CU00825896

Harley Street

A brief history, with notes on nearby
Regent's Park

Harley Street

A brief history, with notes on nearby Regent's Park

John Crawford Adams

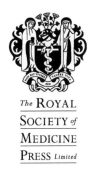

The ROYAL
SOCIETY *of*
MEDICINE
PRESS *Limited*

Published by the Royal Society of Medicine Press Ltd
1 Wimpole Street, London W1G 0AE, UK
Tel: +44 (0)20 7290 2921
Fax: +44 (0)20 7290 2929
Email: publishing@rsm.ac.uk
Website: www.rsmpress.co.uk

British Library Cataloguing in Publication Data
A catalogue record for this book is available from the British Library

---

ISBN 978-1-85315-895-7

Distribution in Europe and Rest of World:
Marston Book Services Ltd
PO Box 269
Abingdon
Oxon OX14 4YN, UK
Tel: +44 (0)1235 465500
Fax: +44 (0)1235 465555
Email: direct.order@marston.co.uk

Distribution in the USA and Canada:
Royal Society of Medicine Press Ltd
c/o BookMasters Inc
30 Amberwood Parkway
Ashland, OH 44805, USA
Tel: +1 800 247 6553 / +1 800 266 5564
Fax: +1 419 281 6883
Email: order@bookmasters.com

Distribution in Australia and New Zealand:
Elsevier Australia
30-52 Smidmore Street
Marrickville NSW 2204, Australia
Tel: +61 2 9517 8999
Fax: +61 2 9517 2249
Email: service@elsevier.com.au

Typeset by Saxon Graphics Ltd
Printed in Europe by the Alden Group, Oxford

Contents

Preface

1. Early beginnings   1
2. Development of the Harley estate (later the Portland estate)   9
3. Arrival of doctors in Harley Street   31
4. Joseph Lister, first medical baron   37
5. The generation after Lister   51
6. A change of character   67
7. Historical notes on the development of Regent's Park   73

Appendix: Lister's 1867 paper on antisepsis   105

Bibliography   111

Index   113

Dedication

My great thanks to Maeve without whose help and encouragement this book could never have been published.

Preface

This book evolved from a long-standing interest in Marylebone and Regent's Park, where I lived for more than thirty years. Harley Street is a central part of the area, and it is interesting to follow its development from fields and pasture land to the elegant street that it became in the Georgian period. For more than a century, the name 'Harley Street' has been famous throughout much of the world, as the centre of British consultative medicine. Its heyday came at the end of the nineteenth century, at a time when specialisation in medicine was gathering pace.

Doctors did not settle in Harley Street in any numbers until about a hundred years after the houses had been built. They were built on the initiative of Edward Harley, later the second Earl of Oxford and Mortimer, whose wife, Henrietta, had inherited the land (part of the Manor of Tyburn) from the Duke of Newcastle. Edward Harley did not live to see the street that bears his name: his plans matured very slowly, and he died almost before construction had got under way. What had begun as the Harley estate thus became the Portland estate, through the marriage of the Harleys' daughter Margaret to the second Duke of Portland.

As Harley Street gradually filled up with doctors, who eventually displaced almost all other residents, the adjacent streets accommodated the overflow, so that Cavendish Square, Wimpole Street and Portland Place acquired the same prestige as Harley Street itself.

This account follows the history of Harley Street, with notes on some of the famous (or infamous) people, lay or medical, who lived either in the street or nearby. Space is devoted in particular to Joseph Lister – later Lord Lister – who by his work on combating wound infection changed the face of surgery. Although most of his epoch-making work was carried out in Scotland, he lived close to Harley Street for the last twenty-five years of his life. Now, in the twenty-first century, he is in danger of being forgotten.

The last chapter is devoted to Regent's Park, which developed during the reign of George IV; it became a favourite place of relaxation for local residents, with the added special interests provided by the zoological gardens, the Colosseum and the Diorama.

The status of Harley Street today is no longer what it was: eminent specialists may now be consulted anywhere, from the hospitals in which they work, to medical clinics or private establishments up and down the country. To be a Harley Street consultant is no longer the prime objective of an aspiring physician or surgeon. Nevertheless, the name still has an indefinable air of eminence.

Chapter 1

Early beginnings

The village of Marylebone and its surrounds

Harley Street came into being, without any medical connections, in the second half of the eighteenth century. Before that, the whole area was pastoral land, with few habitations. The area had never been built up. There was, however, the small village of Marylebone, within the Manor of Tyburn, with its large manor house only a short distance from what would become the north end of Harley Street. The village, earlier known as St Mary-le-Bourn or St Mary-le-Bone, often abbreviated to Marybone, was named after its church, the church of St Mary, and the bourn or stream, known as the Tyburn (Tybourn), that flowed through the fields nearby. This small brook rose in Hampstead and flowed southwards through what is now Regent's Park and across the New Road (now Marylebone Road) to pass through the fields near the site of the present Gloucester Place, before sweeping eastwards close to what is now Blandford Street. Thence it crossed Marylebone High Street to follow the line of the present Marylebone Lane. It crossed the Tyburn Road (now Oxford Street), under a bridge close to the present Stratford Place. It continued southwards, reaching St James's Park and Pimlico before emptying into the Thames near Vauxhall Bridge. In the eighteenth century it was covered in to form a sewer. The stream still flows but it is no longer exposed to view and few people are aware of its existence or its course, or of its having been a picturesque feature of the countryside before the rural scene was overrun by buildings.

The city of London was two miles distant from the village of Marylebone, but there had already been some creeping development westward and north-westward from the city, with some building along the Tyburn Road, later renamed Oxford Street, after the Earl of Oxford and Mortimer.

In Marylebone village itself there had for many years been pleasure gardens that were popular in the summer months, bringing visitors into the village. The gardens, formed in the early part of the seventeenth century from part of the grounds of the original manor house, were reached by a country lane extending northwards from the Tyburn Road. The distance from the Tyburn

Road was less than a mile, but the intervening country, known as Marylebone Fields, was a haunt of robbers and highwaymen, so that well-to-do people visiting the Marylebone gardens would travel by coach, with an armed guard. Lesser people had to ride or walk, and take a chance on getting through without incident.

The facilities available at the gardens were gradually expanded, to the extent that in the eighteenth century they rivalled the better-known pleasure gardens of Ranelagh and Vauxhall. Samuel Pepys had visited the gardens in 1668 and had commented favourably upon them: 'Then we abroad to Marrowbone and there walked in the garden; the first time I ever was there, and a pretty place it is; and here we eat and drank, and stayed till nine at night, and so home by moonlight.' On today's map, the area devoted to the gardens would be represented by a rectangle with its northern boundary extending from the High Street end of Beaumont Street to a point halfway between Devonshire Place and Harley Street, and the southern boundary extending eastwards from a point on the High Street just south of Weymouth Street, almost as far as Harley Street. There was, nearby, a popular retreat known as the Rose Tavern; and a second inn, the Rose of Normandy, spanned the main entrance to the gardens.

The Rose of Normandy was an ancient building even in 1833, when Thomas Smith gave a description of it, and of the bowling green that lay behind it, in his history of Marylebone. At that time it was said to be the oldest house in Marylebone.

> The entrance to this house is by descending a flight of steps, the street having been raised at a later period. It has been repaired at various times, but the original form of the exterior has been preserved, and the staircase and ballusters are coeval with the erection of the building. An extensive yard at the back is laid out as skittle grounds, and is level with the ground floor of the house.

The bowling green at the back of the Rose of Normandy was described in an article in the *Gentleman's Magazine* in 1659:

> The outside a square brick wall, set with fruit trees, gravel walks, 204 paces long, seven broad; the circular walk 485 paces, six broad; the centre square, a bowling green 112 paces one way, 88 another; all except the first double set with quickset hedges, full grown and kept in excellent order and indented like town walls.

By the eighteenth century the bowling green had become part of the Marylebone pleasure gardens.

Rather confusingly, there was a second bowling green close by, on land that had formerly been part of the ground of the manor house, facing the High Street. This bowling green was associated with the other inn, known simply as the Rose

Tavern. This was the meeting place of many of the wilder sort of aristocrats, who used it as a place of gambling.

In the heyday of the Marylebone gardens, at the middle of the eighteenth century, the attractions included refreshments and dining, concerts, theatre, gambling, fireworks, bear-baiting, cock-fighting and prize-fighting, these latter, violent sports being confined to a special area known as the Bear Gardens. The music of George Frideric Handel, who was living in London at the time and who for some years was on the household of the Duke of Chandos, was particularly popular. In 1737 the fee for entrance to the gardens was one shilling, to include refreshments.

After well over a century of popularity the gardens began to decline in the second half of the eighteenth century, as building works in Harley Street and Wimpole Street crept ever nearer from the south. Complaints from nearby residents, who feared for the safety of their properties from the increasingly frequent displays of fireworks in the gardens, led eventually to the compulsory closure of the gardens in 1778, when the site was let to builders. The area was soon to be covered by buildings completing the northward extensions of Harley Street and Wimpole Street.

Close to the Marylebone gardens, in fields near the New Road (Marylebone Road), at what is now the northern extremity of Harley Street, there was a group of allotments used by Protestant (Huguenot) refugees, who had fled from France after the revocation of the Edict of Nantes by Louis XIV in 1685. These refugees had a chapel close to the Marylebone gardens, and near the Rose of Normandy public house. The allotments rented by these Huguenots were often referred to as the French gardens.

Another prominent feature was a large expanse of water, known as the basin (often spelt 'bason'), in the fields near the village of Marylebone, about 150 yards from the south-east corner of the Marylebone gardens. Contemporary maps show it as being about halfway between Cavendish Square and the Marylebone gardens; on a modern map it would be shown approximately in the line of Harley Street. Until it was filled in, it would have blocked any construction of Harley Street and the parallel streets northwards. Figure 1 shows a plan of the area dating from 1746.

The basin was rectangular, 450 feet long and about 130 feet wide. It seems to have been built as a reservoir for the Marylebone Water Company at a time, in the seventeenth century or before, when parts of the city of London received water through pipes (often wooden) and conduits taking water from the Tyburn stream in Marylebone. When this rather meagre source of water was superseded by a more abundant supply, the basin was neglected and it became a local amenity. A sketch by J. B. Chatelain of about 1761 shows it as a small lake, surrounded by vegetation, with people swimming and others strolling along the grassy banks. Contemporary accounts suggest that there were occasional fatalities from drowning in the lake, and there was satisfaction in many quarters when it was finally filled in and built over.

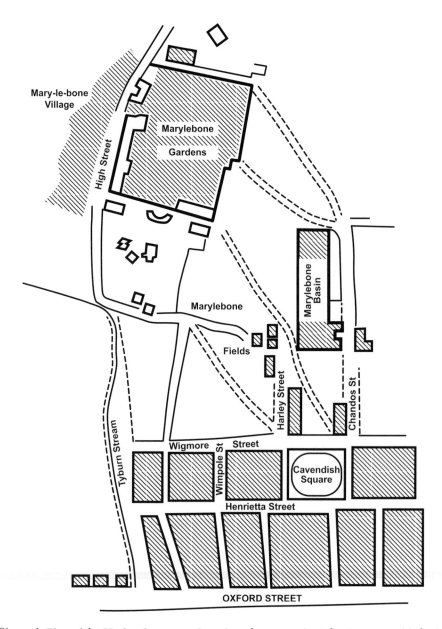

Figure 1 Plan of the Harley Street area based on the survey by John Rocque published in 1746. There has been extensive development along Oxford Street but hardly any along Harley Street and what was to become Wimpole Street. The Marylebone basin is shown midway between Cavendish Square and the Marylebone gardens. Until it was filled in, it blocked any major development along Harley Street. Much of the land between Cavendish Square and Marylebone village still consisted of fields, with open country to the north.

The parish of Marylebone

The wider parish of Marylebone, later to become the Borough of Marylebone before finally being incorporated in Westminster, comprised two ancient manors: the Manor of Tyburn (or Tybourn) and the Manor of Lilestone, each of about 750 acres, or 1500 acres in total. We are concerned here mainly with the Manor of Tyburn, in the fields of which Harley Street and neighbouring streets were to be developed. Both of these ancient manors were described in the Domesday Book. The Manor of Lilestone lay to the west of the Tyburn stream, with its manor house at Lisson Green, near the southern end of the present Lisson Grove. (The old Queen Charlotte's Hospital occupied the site before it was moved to Goldhawk Road.) That manor was later to become the property of the Portman family, and part of it still forms the Portman estate.

The Manor of Tyburn, mainly on the east side of the Tyburn stream, is described in the Domesday Book as part of the ancient demesne of the Abbess and Convent of Barking, who held it under the Crown. The area was rather naively described as being of 'five hides', an inexact measurement, for a hide was the area that could be ploughed by one man in a year. The Manor later came into the ownership of Robert de Vere, second Earl of Oxford, of an earlier creation (distinct from the second Earl of Oxford and Mortimer). In about 1503, in the reign of Henry VII, it was purchased by Thomas Hobson, a merchant, and it passed to another Thomas, probably his son. The Hobsons held it for about forty years. At this point Henry VIII took a liking to the property, the northern part of which, close to the substantial manor house, was well suited to hunting. In 1544, soon after the dissolution of the monasteries, the King 'persuaded' Hobson to exchange the Manor for former church lands near Southampton and on the Isle of Wight. Hobson probably had little option but to accept the King's offer, in the face of what was probably a royal determination to seize the property in any case. (This was truly 'Hobson's choice'.)

Once in possession of the Manor, the King enclosed the northern part with a fence, to form a park for hunting. This became known as Marylebone Park, later to become Regent's Park. The manor house itself, nearby in the old village of Marylebone, was converted into a palace and served as a hunting lodge. The southern parts of the Manor were let to tenants for agriculture.

This arrangement continued until the reign of James I, who in 1611 sold the whole estate, except for the hunting park and certain adjoining pieces, which were retained by the Crown, to Edward Forset (or Forsett) for the sum of £829 3s 4d. Through marriage, the estate subsequently came into the possession of the Austen family. In 1708 Sir John Austen sold it – much reduced in size by the Crown's retention of the hunting park – to John Holles, Duke of Newcastle, for £17,500. The rental value at that time was assessed at £900 per annum.

John Holles, Duke of Newcastle

John Holles, Duke of Newcastle, was the son of Gilbert Holles, third Earl of Clare. He became Member of Parliament for Nottinghamshire and Gentleman of the

Bedchamber to William III. In 1690 he married Margaret Cavendish, daughter and co-heiress of Henry Cavendish, Duke of Newcastle from an earlier creation. There being no male heir when this duke died, John Holles himself received the title of Duke of Newcastle in a fresh creation in 1694. He was a Knight of the Garter and Lord Privy Seal from 1705 until his death in 1711.

John Holles' purchase of the estate, or the Manor of Tyburn, was a landmark event in the history of this part of London. For upon the death of the Duke in 1711 the estate passed to his daughter and sole heiress, Lady Henrietta Cavendish Holles. Henrietta married Edward Harley, son of Robert Harley, Earl of Oxford and Mortimer, and thus the estate, with a large fortune, came into the possession of the Harley family. Almost immediately, Edward Harley and his wife, Henrietta, decided to develop the land as a prestigious district, with high-quality houses designed to attract members of the aristocracy and rich gentry.

The Harley family

The Harley family had originally come from Shropshire, where, in the reign of Edward I (1272–1307), Richard de Harley held the Manor of Harley and repre- sented the county in Parliament. His son Robert, through marriage to the heiress of Brampton, came into possession of Brampton Castle in Herefordshire. A descendant, Thomas Harley of Brampton, born about 1548, received from King James I the honour and castle of Wigmore in Herefordshire, close to Brampton. He died in 1631. His son Robert, born at Wigmore Castle, became Knight of the Bath in 1603 and was appointed Master of the Mint in 1626.

In the Civil War of 1642–51, Robert Harley was on the side of Parliament. His castles at Brampton and Wigmore were besieged, and eventually both were surrendered and burnt, with huge loss of valuables. After Robert's death in 1656, before the restoration of the monarchy, his son Colonel (later Sir Edward) Harley also embraced the side of Parliament; but he later supported the restoration of the monarchy. He was made Governor of Dunkirk (1660–61) and became a Knight of the Bath. He was elected Member of Parliament for Herefordshire in 1646 and 1656, and again after the accession of William III. He died in 1700.

Another of Robert Harley's sons, also Robert, was active in politics and enjoyed a distinguished career, despite serious setbacks. Born in 1661 in Bow Street, London, he became a Whig Member of Parliament for Trigony and later for Radnor, and was Speaker of the House from 1701 to 1705. In a further boost to his career he became Secretary of State in 1704. But in 1708 he suffered the first setback: he had to resign office upon the conviction of his secretary for trea- sonable correspondence with France. He then left the Whig party to become a Tory, determined to undermine the power of the Whigs. He regained his repu- tation, and became Chancellor of the Exchequer and head of a Tory adminis- tration in 1710. In the following year he was attacked with a knife and badly wounded while attending a Committee of the Privy Council in Whitehall. His French assailant, the Marquis de Guiscard, was imprisoned and died soon after- wards in Newgate prison.

After his recovery, Robert Harley was acclaimed in Parliament, and in 1711 Queen Anne rewarded him for his services by advancing him to the peerage as Baron Harley of Wigmore, in the County of Hereford, and Earl of Oxford and Mortimer. As one of the Queen's most trusted ministers, he was appointed Lord High Treasurer of Great Britain in the same year. He was also governor of the South Sea Company, of which he had been a founder. In 1714 fortune turned against him, and he resigned the office of Lord High Treasurer shortly before the Queen died. On the accession of King George I he was impeached by the House of Commons for high treason and specifically for secretly favouring James Stuart, the Old Pretender. He was confined in the Tower of London, but in 1717, after a public trial, he was acquitted by the Lords. He retired from public life and died in 1724.

Apart from his devotion to politics, Robert Harley was noted for the huge collection of manuscripts and books, many devoted to historical matters, that he amassed throughout his lifetime. The manuscripts in this important collection, increased significantly by his son Edward Harley, were eventually to be sold to the British Museum for £10,000, a large sum at the time. As the Harleian Collection they formed a significant part of the Museum's library in its early years. A separate collection of valuable books was sold privately to Thomas Osborne, of Gray's Inn, for £13,000. Their disposal privately was a much lamented loss to the nation.

Robert Harley's son, Edward, was a key player in the development of the Harley estate, which later became the Portland estate. He succeeded to his father's title as second Earl of Oxford and Mortimer in 1724, upon his father's death. His marriage to Henrietta Cavendish Holles, daughter and heiress of the Duke of Newcastle, had taken place in 1713; and soon afterwards the development of the Harley estate began. Like his father, Edward Harley was a serious collector of books and manuscripts, which he housed in a separate building in Marylebone village. After his death the books and manuscripts were sold as part of his father's collection. The substantial building in which they had been stored later became a girls' school at 35 Marylebone High Street.

Unlike his father, Edward Harley avoided any engagement in politics. He was more interested in the arts, and he became a prominent patron of writers and artists. Through his father, however, he had acquired many influential friends and acquaintances among the leading politicians and aristocrats of the time, who would look favourably upon the building developments upon which he was about to embark. Many, indeed, would acquire leases on some of the properties.

Chapter 2

Development of the Harley estate (later the Portland estate)

Early plans

Edward Harley and his wife Henrietta did not lose any time in setting out plans for the development of land bequeathed to Henrietta by the Duke of Newcastle. They instructed their surveyor, John Prince (remembered now by Prince's Street, between Oxford Street and the south-east corner of Cavendish Square), who prepared an ambitious design for the construction of substantial houses in what was to become Cavendish Square (first known as Oxford Square), with a network of streets planned to extend northwards as far as what is now New Cavendish Street (originally Marylebone Street), westwards to Marylebone Lane, and eastwards as far as the present Wells Street. There was also to be a chapel, to be called the Oxford Chapel (later St Peter's on Vere Street), and a market. (The chapel still stands; the market, demolished in 1880, is still recalled by Market Place, just north of Oxford Street, which marks its site.)

Harley's lavish scheme seems to have been inspired by other impressive developments that were in progress in neighbouring parts of London – notably that of Hanover Square, just the other side of Oxford Street. Houses in these new but prestigious areas were being keenly sought by members of the aristocracy and other wealthy citizens anxious to move to this up-and-coming part of London; and the Harleys must have foreseen the possibility of augmenting substantially the large income that they already enjoyed.

Cavendish Square

Building began in Cavendish Square, the first part of the estate to be developed, in 1717; but work proceeded slowly, largely on account of the financial turmoil that followed upon the collapse of the South Sea Company in 1720. So great was this setback that fifty years were to elapse before building in the square was completed. John Prince's planned extension of the new estate northwards to form Harley Street, Wimpole Street and other neighbouring streets – nearly all named after members of the Harley family or their country estates – was begun a few years later; but this project failed to make significant progress until the middle or later years of the eighteenth century, long after Edward Harley had died. Prince's plans were revised in 1720 to speed up the building of the market house (begun in 1720 on the site of the present Market Place) and of the Oxford Chapel, built in 1724. By that time, the earliest buildings on what was then Oxford Square were already occupied. James Gibbs, the architect employed by Edward Harley, himself built three houses in Henrietta Street (now Henrietta Place), and lived in one of them himself. John Prince, the surveyor, also lived in the same street.

The following comment on the building work that was going on in the area is from the *Weekly Medley* of 13 September 1718. It reflects the mood of the populace at the time:

> Round about the New Square [Hanover Square] which is building near Tybourn Road, there are so many other edifices, that a whole magnificent city seems to be risen out of the ground, that one would wonder how it should find a new set of inhabitants. It is said it will be called Hanover Square. On the opposite side of the way towards Mary-le-bone, which seems a higher and finer situation, is marked out a very spacious and noble Square, and many streets that are to form avenues to it. This Square, we hear, is to be called Oxford Square, and that ground has been taken to build houses in it by the Right Honourable Lords, the Earl of Oxford, the Earl of Carnarvon, the Lord Harcourt, the Lord Harley, and several other Noble Peers of Great Britain. The ground sold at first for 2.6d. per foot, afterwards for 15s.

Among the first to take a lease in what was to become Cavendish Square was the Earl of Carnarvon, later the first Duke of Chandos. He leased land which included the whole of the north side of Cavendish Square and extended into the fields some distance to the north. It seems to have been his original intention to build a large mansion as his town house, filling the north side of the square. His main estate was Cannons Park at Edgware, ten miles to the north, and rumour had it that he intended to acquire all the land between his two mansions. If there was anything in this improbable rumour, it came to nothing. In the event he contented himself with building two large wings, one on the north-west corner of the square (at the corner with Harley Street) and the other at the north-east corner (by Chandos Street). The architect for these houses, built in 1724–28, was Edward Shepherd.

Any intention that there may have been to join the two wings by filling in the large intervening area did not materialise: the empty site was left vacant in his time. It was eventually leased, in about 1771, by a Mr Tuffnell, a building speculator, who built a pair of houses in the Palladian style (Numbers 11 and 14), separated by the entrance to Dean's Mews.

The Duke of Chandos himself lived for a time in his house at the north-west corner. Later this substantial house was occupied by Princess Amelia, second daughter of George II. She was to have married the future Frederick the Great of Prussia, but the engagement was broken off for dynastic reasons, and she never married. She was described by a contemporary as a 'horsey, mischief-making woman'. In 1833 the house was in the occupation of Viscount Beresford. The Cavendish Square frontage still stands, but the long extension along Harley Street, containing the domestic offices, has been replaced by six houses.

The other large house built for the Duke of Chandos, at the north-east corner of the square, did not have an important history. In 1833 it was occupied by the Duke of Richmond, but many years ago it was demolished and replaced by a building of no great architectural merit.

In the meantime, other noblemen were moving in elsewhere in Cavendish Square. Simon, Lord Harcourt, a former Tory Lord Chancellor, had a large house built on the east side of the square. He was well known to Edward Harley, for as a prominent lawyer he had obtained the acquittal in 1717 of Harley's father, the first Earl of Oxford and Mortimer, after his impeachment and detention in the Tower of London. Harcourt died in 1727 but the house remained in the family for some years.

Another prominent statesman of the time, Lord Bingley, lived on the west side of the square until his death in 1731. Bingley's house, of distinguished design, filled the greater part of that side of Cavendish Square. Its large garden extended as far as Wimpole Street, where the stables and coach house filled much of the site now occupied by the Royal Society of Medicine. In 1773 the house was bought by Lord Harcourt's grandson, and was known as Harcourt House. In 1825 it came back into the possession of the ground landlord, the fourth Duke of Portland, who lived there for some years, the house shielded from vandals by a high curtain wall and the garden enclosed by a tall screen. The house lasted until 1903, when it was replaced by a block of flats, for which until recently the name Harcourt House was retained.

Thomas Smith in his book *A Topographical and Historical Account of the Parish of St. Mary-le-bone*, published in 1833, records that at the time when he was writing (half a century after most of the houses were built) there were thirty-seven houses in Cavendish Square. (This is confusing, because Horwood's detailed plan of London, published between 1792 and 1799, which marks individual houses, shows only twenty-eight, even though the square appears to be fully built up.) Thomas Smith names all the residents in the square, though not the respective houses in which they lived. The list includes twelve peers, headed by the Duke of Portland, the Duke of Richmond, the Marquis of Titchfield, the Earl of Wicklow and the Earl of Charleville; the other peers were the Lords George Bentinck and Henry Bentinck, Lord Duncannon, Lord Beresford, Lord

Townshend, Lord Dufferin and the Countess of Antrim. There was a generous sprinkling of baronets and knights, and many others of high rank. The inclusion of Sir Martin Shee, President of the Royal Academy of Arts, is a reminder that the area had become popular with artists; writers, too, were well represented. Thomas Smith's list has three medical men: 'S. Love Hammick, surgeon', Dr A. P. W. Philip and Dr John Sims. For a time (1723–38) Number 5 was occupied by Lady Mary Wortley Montagu, a close friend of Lady Henrietta Harley. She left in 1739 to live in Italy. Other notable residents at various times included George Romney, painter, at Number 32, from 1775 to 1797, and Sir Jonathan Hutchinson (1828–1913), surgeon, pathologist and neurologist, at Number 15, from 1874 almost until his death. In the twentieth century, one of the most illustrious residents was Herbert Henry Asquith, first Earl of Oxford and Asquith, long-term Liberal Prime Minister, who lived at Number 20 from 1894 to 1919. Another was Quintin Hogg (1845–1903), founder of the Regent Street Polytechnic, who lived at Number 5 from 1885 to 1898.

In its heyday, at the end of the eighteenth century, Cavendish Square was among the most elegant of London's squares, but it lost most of its notable houses in the course of the twentieth century. The historic houses that remain, some substantially altered, are mostly on the north side of the square, where also now exists, since 1953, Jacob Epstein's statue *Madonna and Child*, suspended on an arch over the entrance to Dean's Mews. The substantial area of grass that fills the centre of Cavendish Square (where sheep once grazed) has been a feature throughout the square's existence. In 1770 there was erected near the middle of the square a statue of the Duke of Cumberland, second surviving son of George II, shown in military uniform and mounted on a large prancing charger. The statue was removed in 1858 but the empty high plinth on which it stood still remains, with the original inscription. A bronze statue by Thomas Campbell of Lord George Bentinck (1802–48), son of the fourth Duke of Portland, erected in 1851, still remains.

Neighbouring developments

The distinguished residents mentioned above all lived in large houses of individual design, contrasting with those in Harley Street and Wimpole Street, which were mainly of uniform size and pattern. There were other individually designed properties close by. Notable among these were Foley House (1758), built for Lord Foley, a cousin of Edward Harley, on the site where the Langham Hotel now stands on Portland Place; and Chandos House, built in 1769–70 by Robert and James Adam for the third Duke of Buckingham and Chandos (grandson of the first Duke of Chandos mentioned above). When they were built, these were both substantial mansions, with large gardens, looking out over unspoilt country. Chandos House remained in the possession of the Chandos family for more than a century. It was later the home of Prince Paul Esterházy, Austrian Ambassador to the Court of St James, for thirty years. The house still stands and has recently been refurbished to a high standard for occupation by the Royal Society of Medicine. But of course the garden has gone and the outlook is now urban.

Also nearby is Portland Place, 'the grandest street in 18th century London'. This was laid out by Robert and James Adam from about 1778 onwards. Like Cavendish Square, it was made up of large houses of individual design, though with some degree of uniformity. A striking and pleasing feature of Portland Place is its great width, which is explained by an undertaking given to Lord Foley by the ground landlord. This stipulated that the view northwards from Foley House would never be obscured by buildings (Figures 2 and 3). The street was therefore made the full width of Foley House, 126 feet. Moreover, Portland Place was not at first a 'through way', for it was closed at the northern end and did not give access to the New Road (Marylebone Road) as it does now.

Foley House blocked the southern end of Portland Place, creating great difficulty for the architect John Nash when he came to design the royal route from Carlton House, the Prince Regent's main residence, to Regent's Park. Nash got over this difficulty by creating an S-shaped curve round Foley House, where Portland Place becomes continuous with Upper Regent Street (see also Figure 4).

Portland Place was a prestigious address and houses there were keenly sought. An early resident was James Holroyd, first Earl of Sheffield, the Whig politician who was largely responsible for the union of England and Ireland in 1801. Other residents listed in 1833 included the Earl of Mansfield, the Earl of Stirling, Viscount Boyle, Lord Walsingham and the Dowager Duchess of Richmond. The site of Number 10, where Admiral Lord Radstock died in 1825, was later to be occupied by Broadcasting House. Field Marshal Lord Roberts lived at Number 47 from 1902 to 1906; the house later became the Polish Embassy. Frances Hodgson Burnett (1849–1924), author of *Little Lord Fauntleroy*, lived at Number 63 from 1893 to 1898. Number 63 was the home of Sir Ralph Milbanke; his daughter Anne Isabella was courted there by Lord Byron. For three years (1863–66) Number 98 was the Embassy of the United States of America, where Henry Brook Adams, the American historian, lived while working for his father, Ambassador Charles Francis Adams.

The Portland estate

Edward Harley did not live to see the completion of his ambitious project. At the time of his death in 1741 the development of Harley Street, Wimpole Street and other neighbouring streets had made little progress. John Rocque's survey, published in 1746 (see Figure 1), showed only scant building northwards from Cavendish Square. The beginnings of Harley Street are shown, with some buildings on one side of the road, but not more than 150 or 200 feet in length. To the north, the Marylebone basin is clearly shown, amid fields. It lies approximately in the line of the future Harley Street, and its position is such that, until filled in, it would have blocked any substantial development of Harley Street northwards. The area between Cavendish Square and Marylebone village, with the Marylebone gardens, is shown still to consist mainly of fields. Most of the development in these early years seems to have taken place in the smaller streets just north of Oxford Street, which have retained their layout to the present.

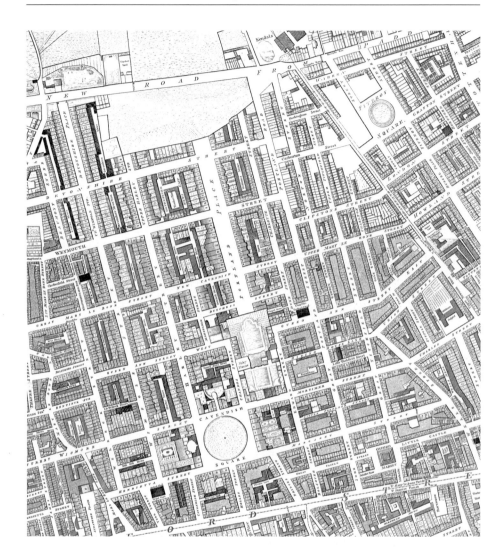

Figure 2 Part of Richard Horwood's detailed plan of London, published in sections between 1792 and 1799. The Portland estate is shown to be now fully built up, except for a small area adjacent to the New Road (Marylebone Road), the last remnant of agricultural land that adjoined the old Marylebone Park. Note the enormous size of Foley House, at the southern end of Portland Place. This blocked any southward extension of Portland Place to link it with Upper Regent Street. When John Nash came to design such a linkage, he had to form an eastern loop of the road (now Langham Place) to circumvent Foley House. (Present-day street names differ in some cases from those on the plan. Thus the north part of Harley Street was formerly known as Upper Harley Street, a name later used to define the extension of Harley Street north of the Marylebone Road. And what was formerly labelled Mary-le-Bone Street is now part of New Cavendish Street.)

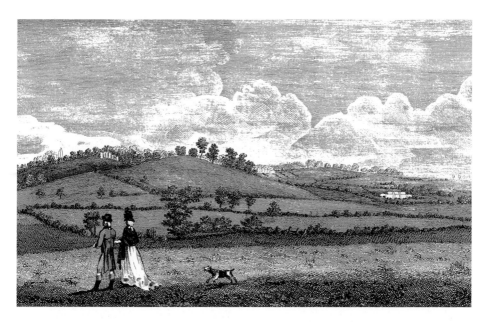

Figure 3 A view included with Horwood's plan of London (1792–99) showing the countryside north of the New Road (Marylebone Road). There had been virtually no building in the fields between Marylebone and Hampstead.

Progress had thus been disappointing, and it was not until much later that the building operations in Harley Street and Wimpole Street were completed, under the supervision – after Harley's death – of successive Dukes of Portland. Horwood's large-scale plan of London, produced in serial parts between 1792 and 1799, shows Wimpole Street to be then fully developed (see Figure 2), as is its northern extension, known then and now as Devonshire Place. The northernmost block of Harley Street, originally known as Upper Harley Street, was still to be completed north of Devonshire Street, as was Portland Place, shown still merging into fields at its northern end. (Rather confusingly, the label Upper Harley Street was later used for the section north of the Marylebone Road.)

On the death of Edward Harley, the manor and estate of Tyburn, by then better known as the Harley estate, passed to the sole heiress, his daughter Lady Margaret Cavendish Harley. Lady Margaret had married the second Duke of Portland in 1734, and thus began the Portland family's ownership of the estate, which became the Portland estate. It remained in the Portland family for four generations, but when in the 1880s the fifth Duke of Portland died without issue, it passed to his sister, Baroness Howard de Walden. Now known as the Howard de Walden estate, though slightly reduced in area, it remains in the ownership of the Howard de Walden family.

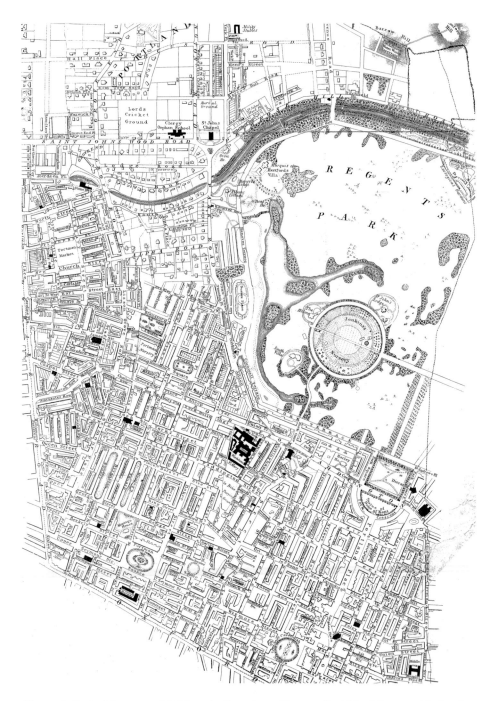

Figure 4 Part of the map of St Mary-le-Bone from Thomas Smith's *A Topographical and Historical Account of the Parish of St. Mary-le-bone* (London: John Smith, 1833).

The Dukes of Portland

The Dukes of Portland originated in the Netherlands, where the family name was Bentinck. William Bentinck was the son of Henry Bentinck, Heer Van Diepenheim, a descendant of a long-established aristocratic family, originally from Overijssel. Born in 1649, he became page of honour in William of Orange's household and was later appointed Gentleman of the Prince's Bedchamber. In 1670 he accompanied William of Orange on a visit to England, and he returned again to England to negotiate with Charles II the marriage of Prince William to Princess Mary, eldest daughter of James, Duke of York (later King James II). This mission was successful and the marriage took place in 1677. Although this was a diplomatic marriage between cousins (Charles I was their common grandfather) it seems to have been reasonably happy.

William Bentinck was deeply involved in preparations for William of Orange's invasion of England in 1688; the Catholic King James II was displaced and William and Mary jointly acceded to the throne by declaration of right. At the invasion Bentinck accompanied the Prince in a thirty-gun frigate. When William and Mary were crowned as joint sovereigns in 1689, Bentinck was created Baron Cirencester, Viscount Woodstock and Earl of Portland. He was Groom of the Stole, First Gentleman of the Bedchamber and Privy Counsellor. He was appointed lieutenant general of the English army and was the most trusted agent of King William's foreign policy. He took part in most of the King's activities in England, Ireland and Flanders. In 1699 he resigned his appointments in the royal household on account of his deep displeasure over the appointment of Arnold Joost van Keppel to certain posts in the household, and his creation as Earl of Albemarle. The two men became implacable enemies; but the Earl of Portland consented still to serve the King in his affairs, and at the time of the King's death in 1702 he was one of those last to speak with him.

The first Earl of Portland died in 1709. His second son, Henry, born in 1682, succeeded to the title of Earl of Portland and to the other titles. In 1716 he was created Marquis of Titchfield and Duke of Portland. He had married, in 1704, Lady Elizabeth Noel, eldest daughter and co-heir of Wriothesley Baptist, Earl of Gainsborough. In 1721 he was appointed Governor of the Island of Jamaica, where he lived until his early death, in 1726, at the age of 44. He was buried at Titchfield, near Southampton, where his wife was also buried in 1736.

Henry and Elizabeth had three sons and seven daughters. William, the elder surviving son, born in 1708, succeeded to the titles, becoming the second Duke of Portland. He travelled for three years in France and Italy and after his return to England he was appointed Lord of the Bedchamber to King George I. In 1734, at the Oxford Chapel in Marylebone, he married Margaret, daughter and heiress of Lord Edward Harley, second Earl of Oxford and Mortimer, and his wife Henrietta; and thus upon Harley's death in 1741 he inherited the Harley estate, then still in an early stage of its development.

The Duke had a distinguished career in his own right. At Windsor in 1740 he received the Order of the Garter from King George II. He was elected a Fellow of the Royal Society (FRS) and was President of the British Lying-in Hospital for Married Women, in Brownlow Street, Long Acre. He was also a trustee of the British Museum. There were two sons of his marriage: William Henry Cavendish Bentinck and Edward Charles Cavendish Bentinck.

William Henry Cavendish Bentinck, born in 1738, became the third Duke of Portland when his father died in 1762. Like other members of his family, he was prominent in politics, being returned as Member of Parliament for Weobly in Herefordshire in 1761. In 1782 he served briefly in Ireland during the Marquis of Rockingham's administration. After this ended, on the death of Rockingham in that year, he served in the Fox/North administration and in 1783 was appointed First Lord of the Treasury. This again was a brief assignment but in 1794 he became Principal Secretary of State for the Home Department in Pitt's government. He was later President of the Council under Addington, and was again First Lord of the Treasury until his death in 1809.

The third Duke of Portland had married, in 1766, Lady Dorothy Cavendish, daughter of William, fourth Duke of Devonshire. Their first son, William Henry Cavendish-Bentinck, born in 1768, inherited the titles, as the fourth Duke of Portland. He added Scott, his wife's maiden name, to his own name by permission of King George III. He was Lord Lieutenant of the County of Middlesex. His wife was Henrietta Scott, daughter of General Scott. They had nine children, of whom the first, William Henry Cavendish Bentinck-Scott, born in 1800, inherited the titles on the death of the fourth Duke in 1854.

As the fifth Duke and last in the line, William Cavendish Bentinck-Scott lived a lonely, semi-reclusive life. He had been rejected by a lady whom he loved, the attractive opera singer Adelaide Kemble, and he never married. He spent much of his time at Welbeck Abbey, his large estate in Nottinghamshire, and came infrequently to his London house in Cavendish Square. Immensely wealthy, he led a way of life that became eccentric: at Welbeck Abbey he had the furniture removed from most of the rooms and had the walls painted pink. Neglecting the main house, he employed scores of men to dig an extensive network of tunnels and underground rooms. These included a library, a huge billiards room with space for twelve tables and a vast subterranean ballroom. This was strange, for the Duke seems to have disliked being part of a large company, and when travelling in his carriage in London he would often keep the blinds drawn. He took only a small part in public life: he served as Member of Parliament for King's Lynn from 1824 to 1826, and he was Deputy Lieutenant of Nottinghamshire from 1859 to 1879. When he died, childless, in 1879, the Portland estate passed to his sister, Baroness Howard de Walden, and became the Howard de Walden estate. This now comprises most of the property bequeathed to Henrietta Cavendish Holles by the Duke of Newcastle in 1708. It includes the whole of Harley Street except for the northernmost terrace on the east side, which is part of the Crown

Estate, and other houses in the southernmost terrace, adjacent to Cavendish Square.

Harley Street, Wimpole Street and the cross streets

As mentioned above, whereas the houses in Cavendish Square, the first part of Edward Harley's project to be started, were mostly large and of individual design (see Figures 5 and 6), bespoken by members of the aristocracy and rich gentry, those in Harley Street, Wimpole Street and the adjacent lesser streets – nearly all named after members of the Harley family or after their country estates – were typically of uniform size and design, with differences mainly in detail, especially of the interiors. Plots of land were let out on long leases to speculative builders or, in some cases, to individuals. All the houses conformed to the prevailing Georgian style.

Most prominent among the architects instructed was James Gibbs (1682–1754), who was also responsible, among other projects, for the famous church of St Martin's in the Fields in Trafalgar Square, the Radcliffe Camera in Oxford, the Senate House in Cambridge and St Bartholomew's Hospital in London. Gibbs was born in Aberdeen and had studied in Italy. A disciple of Sir Christopher Wren, he was for a time one of the commissioners for building new churches in London, until he was dropped on account of his Roman Catholicism. Gibbs supervised the general architectural features of the houses to be built, and he lived himself in one of his own three houses in Henrietta Street (now Henrietta Place). Other architects – mainly for the later houses – included John Johnson, W. Thomas Collins and, for at least one house, the illustrious James Wyatt (1746–1813).

Gibbs stipulated the use of red and grey stock bricks. The window arches could be straight or compass (curved), and the jambs could be of rubbed brick or stone. A feature of the ornamentation on many of the houses was the use of keystones in the door arches faced with a representation of the head of a bearded man (Figure 7), such as were listed in the Coade catalogue of the period and were to be found in other parts of London. Many such keystones are still preserved in Harley Street and elsewhere.

The road level at the front of the houses was raised by several feet by earth removed to form the basements. This is evident today from the downward slope to the mews behind the houses, which did not have basements. Virtually every house had its mews premises at the back, with stable and coach house, and rooms for the groom or coachman above. It is noticeable still that in many cases the coach-house doors were unusually high compared with those constructed in later times. Extra height was necessary to allow easy access for the high coaches that were common in the eighteenth and nineteenth centuries.

The houses in Harley Street and Wimpole Street were of only moderate size for the period, though they would be considered large as town houses today. They were all terraced rather than detached. The ground floor was raised above road level usually by four to six steps, to allow reasonable light to the basement. A wrought iron balcony at first-floor level usually ran the full width of the house.

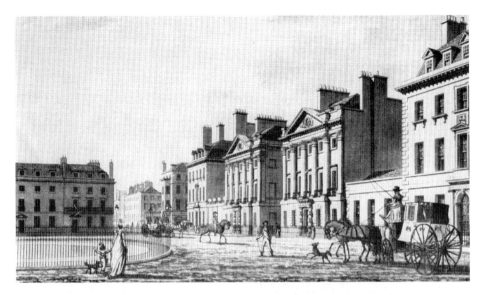

Figure 5 Cavendish Square in the early nineteenth century. The view is of the north side of the square, with the right turn into Harley Street just in front of the four-storey building just left of centre. From G. Mackenzie, *Marylebone* (London: Macmillan, 1972).

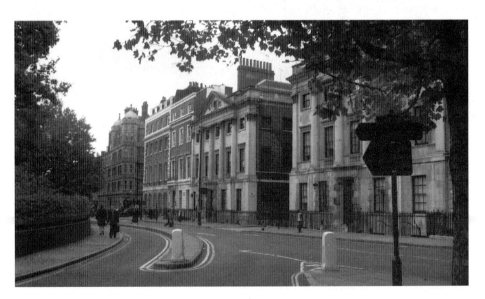

Figure 6 Cavendish Square today. Many of the buildings on the north side of the square have survived. The prominent gap between the twin buildings just right of centre is the entrance to Dean's Mews, spanned by a bridge upon which is suspended Epstein's sculpture *Madonna and Child* (not shown). The Harley Street turning is next on the right beyond Dean's Mews.

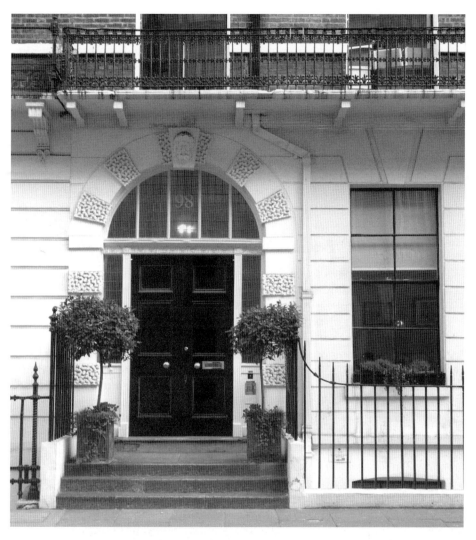

Figure 7 A typical Harley Street house. On the keystone in the door arch is a representation of the face of a bearded man. The ground floor is slightly raised, allowing some light to the basement. The balcony extends across the full width of the house.

The front door was wide, with a fanlight above. It opened into a spacious hall giving onto two large rooms, one facing the road and the other facing the rear. These reception or living rooms were confined to one side of the house, as was usual with terraced houses: on the other side of the hall was the party wall shared with the adjoining house. Further down, the hall narrowed to a corridor leading to one or two small rooms at the back of the house.

From the entrance hall a staircase gave access to the first floor, with large rooms broadly matching those on the ground floor, and a smaller room over the entrance hall. The larger rooms, one of which would normally be the (with)drawing room, would often be finely decorated. Further stairs led up to the second floor, and beyond that to the attic floor, where in most cases the domestic staff would be accommodated. The basement was reached by a narrow staircase from the rear part of the entrance hall. Here were sited the large kitchen and a number of smaller rooms that completed the domestic offices. There might be a small garden or yard behind the house, with access at the back to the mews premises.

Although nearly all the houses conformed to this general pattern, there were often variations of design. In many houses the interiors were fitted out to a high standard, with fine staircases and painted ceilings. Outside, at the road frontage, the better houses were furnished with handsome wrought iron lamp holders, often supported on a wrought iron arch over the steps, and the fanlight over the door was often pleasingly decorated.

Houses in Harley Street were similar to other substantial houses of the period in many parts of London. They were less elegant than those in Cavendish Square and Portland Place, but very comfortable for the principals, if not for the servants, who often had to put up with dingy quarters in the basement or attic, with few amenities or comforts.

As in most London houses of the period, drainage was at first into a cesspit beneath the house or beneath its tiny back yard or garden. Sewage was often collected at night. This system of drainage changed radically after 1875, when Sir Joseph Bazalgette (1819–91) completed his enormous project for a comprehensive system of drainage for the whole of London. He oversaw the construction of large sewers at three levels, leading out finally through drains on both sides of the Thames to processing plants eleven miles east of London. With the inception of this system of main drainage, the use of cesspits was soon prohibited.

In general, a supply of piped water was already available when the houses were built, but at first it was brought only to the basement. Servants had the unenviable task of carrying large jugs of water upstairs from the basement for their employers to use on the upper floors. Fitted bathrooms were a luxury that gained favour only after the middle of the Victorian era.

Heating of the houses was still by coal fires and there were open cooking ranges in the basement kitchen. In the earliest of the Harley Street houses, lighting was still by candles or oil lamps. Candles were expensive and oil lamps potentially dangerous. Both contributed enormously to the dirt that gathered remorselessly in every house. The atmosphere was laden with smoke from countless chimneys, domestic and industrial. This was a nightmare for the mistress of the house and for the servants, who had the task of trying to keep things clean. The grime-laden air infiltrated every recess in every room of the house. With an often smoking fire grate as well, and several candles or lamps burning at the same time, it became impossible to keep any room clean for more than a few hours.

Those houses that were built after the first decade of the nineteenth century were likely to have had gas lighting installed at the time of construction. If not, most would have gas laid on within a few years, for gas was widely available after about 1810. It was expensive at first but it was convenient and relatively safe if due precautions were taken. Gas gradually decreased in cost, so that by the middle of the nineteenth century it was cheaper than candles or oil lamps. Unless handled with great care, however, it was still messy: used carelessly, it could add black smoke to the atmosphere and thus it did not immediately solve the problem of black dirt settling on any horizontal surface. The introduction of incandescent mantles added greatly to the intensity of gaslight and also reduced the smoke. Lighting by electricity did not become common until the end of the nineteenth century – more than a hundred years after most of the houses in Harley Street had been built. When it came, it was of course a huge boon, not only because of its convenience but also on account of its cleanliness. It also permitted greater intensity of illumination, enabling those who wished to read or write after dark to do so in comfort. The use of gas for cooking did not come until much later: the open coal-fired range continued in use until the end of the Victorian era and beyond.

Residents in the Harley Street area were well served, so far as general amenities and purchase of essentials were concerned. As the houses on the estates went up, Oxford Street was developing into a prestigious shopping zone, with numerous brightly lit shops that remained open until a late hour, as well as a good sprinkling of public houses. (Harley Street's own pub, the Turk's Head, at Number 51, established in about 1847, failed to flourish and closed after only three years.) The Oxford Market had been built in 1724, a little to the east of Cavendish Square. There was some delay before it could be opened, because of objections from Lord Craven, who feared that it would offer harmful competition to his own Carnaby Market, close by on the other side of Oxford Street: it was not until 1731 that the Oxford Market came into full service. Its design, by James Gibbs, was similar to that of many markets in country towns, with an arcaded ground floor. The steep roof was surmounted by a cupola, with weather vane above. It was a pleasant building but seemingly the market was not a great success commercially. It survived for 150 years but was pulled down in 1880.

Residents' religious needs were served initially by the Oxford Chapel (renamed St Peter's, on Vere Street, in 1832), built in 1724 a mere hundred yards from the south-west corner of Cavendish Square. Also designed by James Gibbs, it was a plain Georgian-style building with an elegant interior: a much smaller forerunner of Gibbs's later masterpiece of St Martin's in the Fields. The building still stands but it is no longer used for church services. In its earlier years the chapel saw many prestigious ceremonies, notably the wedding in 1734 of Lord and Lady Harley's daughter Margaret (their only child) to the second Duke of Portland.

Residents in the more northerly parts of the estate had for many years had the choice of attending the tiny church of St Mary in Marylebone High Street (Figure

8). Built in 1741 to replace a fifteenth-century church on the same site, it was much too small for its purpose; but it was not until 1817 that it was eventually replaced by the fine new parish church, designed by Thomas Hardwick, facing the York Gate entrance to Regent's Park on the Marylebone Road. The ancient church of St Mary survived for some years after being superseded by the new parish church, and was known as the old parish chapel. In 1949 it was declared unsafe and was demolished, but its site is preserved as a garden of rest.

After 1824 another popular place of worship was John Nash's elegant church of All Souls in Langham Place (Figure 9). The church itself still has elegance, but its visual appeal has been compromised by tall buildings on nearly every side, including the rebuilt Langham Hotel, St George's Hotel and Broadcasting House.

This was a time of large church congregations and active church building programmes, and a further church was built on the north side of the Marylebone Road, little more than 200 yards from Thomas Hardwick's new parish church on the south side of the road (Figure 10). This was Trinity Church, on the corner with Albany Street. Designed by Sir John Soane, who had recently completed designs for the Bank of England, it was unusual in facing south, with the altar at

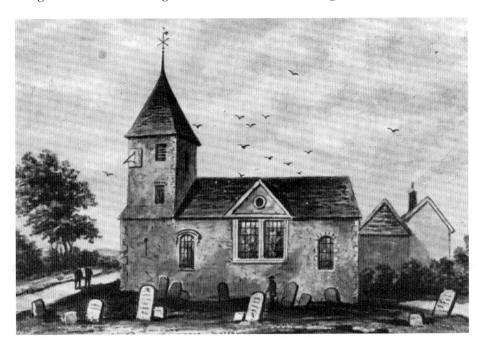

Figure 8 Church of St Mary in Marylebone village, built in 1401. This church was replaced by another on the same site in 1740, which in turn was replaced by the present Marylebone parish church, opened in 1817, on the Marylebone Road. The site of the church of St Mary was retained and converted to a garden of rest, still a feature of Marylebone High Street.

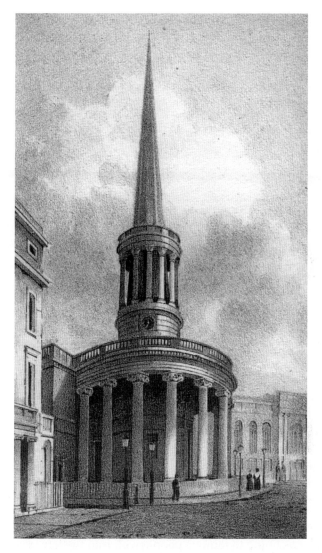

Figure 9 Church of All Souls, Langham Place. Designed by John Nash and consecrated in 1824, it was only a short walk from Harley Street and was a popular place of worship among residents of the Portland estate. From Thomas Smith's *A Topographical and Historical Account of the Parish of St. Mary-le-bone* (London: John Smith, 1833).

the north end. It is a handsome building with the portico raised on a shallow plinth and featuring four ionic columns surmounted by a Grecian frieze. The tower is in two storeys, the first square, and the upper storey round, with six columns surmounted by a cupola. The church is no longer used for church services but has other ecclesiastical functions.

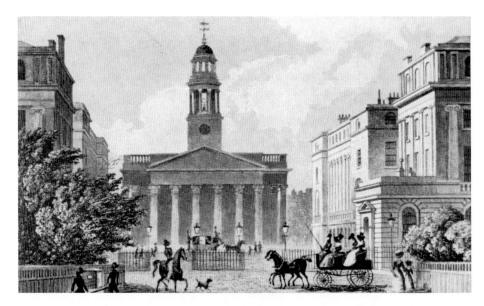

Figure 10 The parish church and York Gate on Marylebone Road, designed by Thomas Hardwick to replace the old church of St Mary on Marylebone High Street. The new church came into use in 1817. From *Regent's Park: A study of the development of the area from 1086 to the present day* by Ann Saunders (Devon: David & Charles, 1969).

Population of Marylebone

With the development of networks of new streets throughout Marylebone in the second half of the eighteenth century, there was an enormous and rapid increase in the population of the parish. Recorded as only 5,000 for the whole parish in 1740, the population had increased to 64,000 by 1891, and there was a relentless further expansion throughout the twentieth century.

Distinguished early residents

Harley Street was home to famous people well into the later years of the nineteenth century. In the early years there was no special connection with the medical profession. Well over a century elapsed after the first houses had been built before doctors began to arrive in any numbers. Instead, houses were taken by wealthy individuals of substantial rank, by artists and writers, by naval and army officers, active or retired, and even by distinguished politicians. Given that building operations were continuing throughout most of the eighteenth century and beyond, with inevitable chaos in the streets and uncontrollable dust and dirt, as well as frequent crime, these early residents might be thought bold indeed to have moved in while development was still proceeding all around them.

Prominent among the artists who came early to reside in Harley Street was Allan Ramsay (1713–84), son of the Scottish poet of the same name. After studying in Italy, he became a distinguished portrait painter, acclaimed by Horace Walpole as superior to Joshua Reynolds as a painter of women. In 1767 he became portrait painter to George III. He lived at 67 Harley Street (now Number 45) in a house that has become part of the present Queen's College. Ramsay was a noted conversationalist and an active member of Samuel Johnson's circle.

A later artist resident was J. M. W. Turner (1775–1851), who lived at 64 Harley Street from 1804 to 1808 before moving round the corner to 23 Queen Anne Street. Thereafter he lived largely by the Thames in Twickenham, and later in Chelsea, but he retained the house in Queen Anne Street as a private gallery, studio and part-time residence, cared for by his long-term retainer Hannah Danby. In contrast to Allan Ramsay, Turner was a somewhat eccentric, secretive man, highly intelligent but far from gregarious.

This part of London was popular among artists in general, with many living further east towards Charlotte Street, where John Constable lived for many years. In the twentieth century, however, it was gradually superseded by Chelsea as the favoured quarter for artists.

Another famous non-medical resident in Harley Street was Sir Arthur Wellesley (1769–1852), later Lord Wellington, who lived at Number 11 after his return from India and his marriage to Lady Katherine Pakenham. He left in 1808 to conduct the Peninsular War campaign of 1808–14. He was not the only high-ranking service chief to live in Harley Street. Alexander Hood (1726–1814), later Admiral Hood and in 1800 created Viscount Bridport, lived at Number 7 (now 16). Admiral Lord Keith (George Elphinstone) (1746–1823), who married Esther Thrale, Dr Johnson's little favourite, known as Queenie when she was a girl in Streatham, lived at Number 45 (now 89).

Lord Nelson's widow lived in Harley Street after her husband's death at Trafalgar in 1805, and died there. Lady Rodney, widow of Admiral Lord Rodney, also moved to Harley Street after Rodney's death in Hanover Square in 1792.

Of the politicians who lived in Harley Street, the most famous was William E. Gladstone (1809–98), son of Sir John Gladstone, a Liverpool merchant. William was Member of Parliament first for Newark and later for Oxford University and finally for Midlothian. He used 73 Harley Street between his terms of office as Prime Minister. A fine parliamentary debater, first a Conservative but later a Liberal, he oversaw the introduction of the first national system of education ever to be established in England. He served four separate terms as Prime Minister, until age eventually caught up with him, causing him to resign in 1894 at the age of eighty-five. It is recorded that on one occasion, in 1878, an angry mob surged down Harley Street and smashed windows at Gladstone's house, in protest against his opposition to the pro-Turkish policy of Benjamin Disraeli, then Prime Minister, who enjoyed the strong support of the public. This fiery demonstration is a reminder that the Victorian period had its full share of mob violence.

Gladstone's house at 73 Harley Street had previously been occupied by Sir Charles Lyell, the geologist, whose *Principles of Geology* significantly influenced the scientists of the day.

A blue plaque at 90 Harley Street (previously 1 Upper Harley Street) commemorates Florence Nightingale (1820–1910), the iron-willed reformer of nursing practice and hygiene, who was living there in 1853, before her departure for the Crimea in 1854 with thirty-eight nurses. She had previously taken charge, as superintendent, of the Hospital for Invalid Gentlewomen in Chandos Street, and had promptly transferred the establishment to what was then Upper Harley Street. On her return in 1856 she was rightly fêted for her immense services to nursing, which had hugely reduced the death toll among wounded soldiers. A fund of £50,000 was subscribed to enable her to establish a training institute for nurses at St Thomas's Hospital and King's College Hospital. She received the Order of Merit in 1907, when she was near the end of her long life.

One of the few other blue plaques in Harley Street commemorates Sir Arthur Wing Pinero (1855–1934), the actor who became a popular playwright in the dramatists' heyday of the 1890s, along with Oscar Wilde, Bernard Shaw and others. Initially concerned mainly with farce, he later wrote plays that dealt with social problems, notably *The Second Mrs. Tanqueray* and *Trelawny of the 'Wells'*.

Not in Harley Street itself, but on the fringe, in Welbeck Street, lived the eccentric Lord George Gordon (1751–93), activator of the Gordon Riots of 1780. The Eton-educated aristocrat had retired from the Royal Navy as a lieutenant at the age of 21, and became a Member of Parliament two years later. As leader of a Protestant association and an outspoken opponent of Catholicism, he had opposed the passage in 1778 of a Bill for the relief of Catholics from certain burdensome restrictions. The passage of the Bill sparked intense anger among Protestants, and in 1780 Gordon directed a march upon the House of Commons by 50,000 protesters, demanding repeal of the Act. Serious rioting followed, and lasted five days, until troops were eventually called out. Before the violence ended, more than 259 people had been killed and a huge amount of property had been destroyed. Gordon was charged with high treason but, surprisingly, he was acquitted. Thereafter he embraced the Jewish faith and grew a long, flowing beard. In 1787 he was convicted for libelling Marie Antoinette, Queen of France, and was committed to Newgate prison, where he died from gaol fever at the age of forty-two.

This was a major tragedy. But Harley Street saw tragedy on its doorstep on at least two other occasions: tragedies that doctors living nearby were powerless to avert. These incidents are recorded by Thomas Smith in his 1833 *history of Marylebone*. The first incident related to a wealthy banker, living in what was then called Upper Harley Street (now the upper end of Harley Street itself):

> Died at his house in this street, June 21, 1800, in consequence of a melancholy accident, which he met with on the preceding night, William Bosanquet Esq. He had been making some alterations in his

house, and, among others, had removed the balcony from his back drawing room window: unfortunately forgetting this circumstance, he walked out, and immediately fell into the area, and, in his fall, broke the vertebrae of his back, and was otherwise severely bruised and injured. He was sensible of his inevitable dissolution, and bore his sufferings with a fortitude almost unparalleled; dictating, in the extremity of torture, some additions to his will. He left a most amiable lady, and ten children, to deplore his loss....

The second incident occurred on 27 April 1831, two years before Thomas Smith's book was published. This was at the house of Lord Walsingham, which at two o'clock in the morning was discovered to be on fire. Lord Walsingham was burnt to death in his bed chamber; and Lady Walsingham, in her fright, 'precipitated herself out of the window of her room, on to some leads at the back of the house, and shortly after expired, from the injuries she had received'. Almost as an after-thought, Smith gives a full list of the residents in the street. This was at the time when the houses were occupied by elite gentry, with a sprinkling of peers and high-ranking army officers; no mention is made of any member of the medical professional. Evidently at that time doctors had not yet moved in.

Chapter 3

Arrival of doctors in Harley Street

Early practices

Medical men did not begin to settle in Harley Street and the adjacent streets much before the middle of the nineteenth century. That was more than a hundred years after the earliest houses had been built. As late as the 1860s there were not more than a dozen or so doctors practising there. But the trend was set: by 1873 there were thirty-six doctors with Harley Street addresses, and numbers were increasing rapidly. Even so, doctors were still greatly outnumbered by private residents.

One of the first men to make a fortune from his practice in Harley Street brought the street into disrepute rather than setting a good example. This was John St John Long, a personable Irishman who had studied art in Dublin before venturing into the field of medicine. He does not seem to have had a proper medical training, but he had a personality that in large measure made up for this omission. It was as early as 1828 when he set up in practice at Number 41 Harley Street (now 84). Through his enviable good looks and charming manner he soon attracted patients – especially fashionable ladies with little the matter with them other than boredom and a desire to be pampered. Some no doubt had genuine illnesses, but others had imaginary ones that took them to this attractive physician. Such fame did he enjoy throughout London that the street outside his house was liable to be jammed with carriages waiting upon these fragile women. The patients were often treated in groups. A favourite method of treatment was by inhalations, through long pink tubes. Afterwards there might be a session of massage. With so many patients, and with treatment no doubt at a high cost, Long was said to be earning £10,000 a year – a large income at the time. In reality he was no more than a quack: eventually, indeed, he was dubbed 'the king of quacks'.

John St John Long's luck ran out after a few years, when two young female patients died while under his care, within a short time of each other. It is not clear exactly why they died; but Long was charged with manslaughter in each case, and in one he was convicted. He was lucky to escape with a surprisingly light sentence – a fine of £250. But his practice was broken. Before long he died from tuberculosis, at the age of only thirty-five.

The story of John St John Long marked an unfortunate beginning to the slow invasion of Harley Street by more reputable physicians and surgeons, who came in increasing numbers in the second half of the nineteenth century and the early years of the twentieth century. There was no particular reason why Harley Street should have been chosen by doctors as a place in which to practise. It has to be assumed that they came there for no other reason than to live in a prestigious area among well-to-do people, some of whom might need their services. There was also the fact that the City of London, where many doctors had traditionally practised close to the great teaching hospitals – notably Guy's and St Bartholomew's (Barts) – was losing its appeal as a place of residence. People were moving outwards, and new teaching hospitals were being built west of the City, on the borders of the countryside: these included the Middlesex Hospital, University College Hospital, the Charing Cross Hospital, St George's Hospital and St Mary's.

After a big reputation had been made by a few early specialists, others saw the advantage of mixing with the elite. Before their move to Harley Street, doctors had often favoured an address close to the fashionable residential area centred on Piccadilly where, in Dover Street, Lord and Lady Harley themselves had chosen to live, rather than in their Harley estate in Marylebone. Savile Row was one such street, highly favoured for a time. But there was no fixed pattern. John Hunter (1728–93), the famous surgeon, researcher and comparative anatomist, had lived first in Jermyn Street but later built a large house in Leicester Square. Even during the heyday of Harley Street, at the turn of the nineteenth/twentieth century, there were many eminent physicians and surgeons who lived and practised elsewhere in London. The vicinity of the great squares that had recently been built – Hanover Square, Berkeley Square, Portman Square and particularly Manchester Square – was especially favoured, and anywhere in present-day Mayfair was regarded as a good address from which to practise.

Specialist practice

The doctors coming to Harley Street tended to be specialists rather than general doctors: they included ophthalmologists, laryngologists, gynaecologists and paediatricians, as well as general surgeons and physicians. Although it is now regarded as essential that consultants should gain skill in narrow fields of medicine and surgery, specialisation was often frowned upon in the nineteenth century as being unnecessary: a physician or surgeon – so it was thought – should be able to cover the whole field. The medical press was largely sympathetic to that view, which was, however, gradually to change as the twentieth century dawned.

At the time when specialists began to take houses in Harley Street, it is clear that only a few of the scores of men – and the occasional woman – who sat behind their desks in elegant consulting rooms possessed ability and skill to match their outward show of eminence. Many had no special talent and there must have been more than a few charlatans, keen to cash in on the big reputation that Harley Street was earning. A later consultant, Dr Ernest Jones, candidly recalling early memories of Harley Street, wrote:

> What a closed corporation, like an expensive club, the consulting world of those days was, where everyone gossiped with the other and looked askance at anyone who was not quite the thing. And many of them were intellectually very inferior people.

Among the earliest reputable men to practise in or adjacent to Harley Street, at 3 Cavendish Place (just round the corner from Harley Street, off Cavendish Square), was Joseph Clover (1825–82), remembered as a pioneer anaesthetist when anaesthesiology was a science in its infancy. Chloroform and ether were the main anaesthetic agents, generally inhaled directly from a gauze-covered face mask. Clover designed new methods of administering these noxious agents, one still remembered as 'Clover's bag', from which the patient inhaled the vapour. Among his patients at one time or another were Florence Nightingale, Sir Robert Peel and Emperor Napoleon III (see below). After his death, a biennial lectureship was established in his honour at the Royal College of Surgeons of England.

Close by, at 15 Cavendish Square, lived Sir Jonathan Hutchinson (1828–1913), a surgeon at the London Hospital and a prolific writer. He was a notable scientist, elected a Fellow of the Royal Society. Though prominent as Professor of Surgery at the London Hospital and sometime President of the Royal College of Surgeons of England, he was also renowned as an ophthalmologist and more particularly as a specialist in venereal disease (a wide range of specialties for one man to embrace, even in the nineteenth century). Syphilis was common at the time, and Hutchinson is said (perhaps rather incredibly) to have seen a million cases. He is remembered for having described the three primary features of congenital syphilis: notched incisor teeth, interstitial keratitis and sclerosis of the eardrum. This combination of abnormal features later became known as Hutchinson's triad.

One of the most stylish and successful surgeons of the early period was Sir Henry Thompson, Bart (1820–1904), who lived at 35 Wimpole Street. Practising largely in the pre-Listerian age, before the introduction of the aseptic (safe) techniques of surgery, his scope for major surgery was limited. Nevertheless, he made a name for himself as a urologist. His reputation was enhanced enormously when he treated King Leopold of the Belgians for vesical calculus (bladder stone). An expert with the lithotrite (a special instrument, inserted through the urethra, for crushing bladder stones), he was able to grasp the stone and to crush it. 'My blades were full: I screwed home tight and withdrew them filled with a good quantity of phosphoric debris.' Among his patients at various times were Charles Dickens (a resident of Marylebone but one who was critical of the local architecture) and William Makepeace Thackeray. Later he was called to treat Emperor Napoleon III, then living in exile in England. With Dr Clover as anaesthetist, Thompson operated to remove a urinary obstruction, the nature of which was not disclosed. In this case things went tragically wrong. As he related: 'A sudden change occurred, and death without pain took place at 10.45'. The cause of the Emperor's death is unclear: perhaps it was related to the anaesthetic. Thompson was a versatile man who painted well enough to exhibit at the Royal Academy, wrote novels and studied astronomy in his own observatory. He was noted for the 'octave' dinners that he gave regularly at his house, for eight guests, at eight o'clock, with eight courses. On his guest list were many famous people, including on occasion the Prince of Wales (later King George IV) and Sir Arthur Conan Doyle, who for a time lived at 2 Devonshire Place, nearby. Thompson lived just long enough to enjoy briefly the new luxury of motoring.

It was probably only through coincidence that Dr George Harley (1829–96), another of the early group of specialists, came to live and practise in Harley Street, at Number 25. He seems not to have been related to Edward Harley, Earl of Oxford. Nevertheless, he was a man of talent in his own right – enough of a scientist to be elected, in 1865, a Fellow of the Royal Society. After qualifying in medicine in Edinburgh and holding junior posts as house physician and house surgeon at the Edinburgh Royal Infirmary, he studied physiology and chemistry in Paris and was President of the Parisian Medical Society in 1853. Settling finally in London, he became Lecturer on Practical Physiology and Histology at University College in 1855. He was elected a Fellow of the Royal College of Physicians of Edinburgh, and later became Professor of Medical Jurisprudence at University College in London, and physician to University College Hospital (1860). He experimented with anaesthetics, at great risk to himself. In 1887 he also demonstrated a machine that reproduced sound recorded on a grooved wax plate – a forerunner of the gramophone. Perhaps intrigued by Sir Henry Thompson's octave dinners, he arranged regular Sunday breakfasts for ten or twelve guests, attended at times by celebrities who included Charles Dickens, Sir Edwin Landseer and the caricaturist George Cruikshank.

Like ophthalmology, laryngology was a field in which specialisation began early. Sir Morell Mackenzie (1837–92) was one such specialist, with a flourishing practice at first in Harley Street and later in Cavendish Square. (This suggests that in Mackenzie's time even Harley Street was not quite 'good enough' for the top people: Cavendish Square was the apex of the pyramid.) Mackenzie came into disfavour towards the end of his life because of a controversy with German laryngeal surgeons over the plight of the German Crown Prince Frederick, husband of Queen Victoria's eldest daughter, also Victoria. Called to Berlin to advise on the Crown Prince's throat complaint, Mackenzie wrongly suspected that the diagnosis might be syphilis, whereas in fact it turned out to be laryngeal cancer, which proved fatal in 1888, shortly after the Prince had become Emperor Frederick III. Not surprisingly, the German surgeons were upset and angered by this slur on the Crown Prince's integrity and by Mackenzie's delay in reaching a clear diagnosis; and the new ruler of Germany, Kaiser Wilhelm II, was deeply offended. The incident attracted huge publicity among a populace that was keenly interested in anything medical, and especially in anything that touched upon the aristocracy or royalty. Mackenzie later wrote a book about the incident, which made matters worse. He was censured by the Royal College of Surgeons of England, and the incident cast a shadow for a while over Harley Street's reputation. Nevertheless, Mackenzie, who died four years later, was well regarded as a laryngologist, and had been jointly instrumental in the foundation in 1863 of the Hospital for Diseases of the Throat in London's Golden Square. He was also possibly the first to issue a warning, in the *Strand Magazine*, of a link between tobacco smoking and cancer.

Chapter 4

Joseph Lister, first medical baron

Surgical revolution

Because of his epoch-making work on combating wound infection, Joseph Lister (1827–1912) marks a watershed between hazardous, almost primitive surgery and safer, definitive surgery that became possible only after his work had been fully accepted and assimilated. Before Lister's time, operations upon the human body were so dangerous, on account of wound infection, that they were avoided whenever possible. Abdominal surgery as we know it today had hardly begun, because of the high risk of fatal wound infection. In the post-Listerian era, operative surgery became increasingly safe and it went from strength to strength.

Fortuitously, Lister's brilliant work followed closely upon the introduction of methods of anaesthetising patients, initially by the inhalation of ether. The credit for the introduction of anaesthetics goes jointly to two Americans, Crawford Long (1815–78), of Athens, Georgia, who was the first to use ether in 1842 but who delayed publication of his observations for seven years; and to W. T. G. Morton (1819–68), of Boston, Massachusetts, whose use of ether anaesthesia was reported in 1846. The use of anaesthetic agents in itself was a huge landmark in the evolution of surgical practice; but it did nothing to combat the scourge of devastating wound infection, which was the prime bar to any advance in operative surgery. It is interesting that Lister was present as a student when the first operation ever to be carried out in England under ether anaesthesia was undertaken, by Robert Liston at University College Hospital in London on 21 December 1846.

Of Lister it may be said truthfully that he revolutionised surgery. Indeed, it has been claimed that his contribution to surgery was greater than that of any other man. Safe operative surgery may be said to have begun only after the assimilation of Lister's work (1867), and it has thus been practised for little more than 140 years.

Early life

Lister lived in London for the last thirty-four years of his life, at 12 Park Crescent, just round the corner from the north end of Harley Street (Figure 11). He was to this extent a 'Harley Street surgeon', even though his most definitive work had been carried out in Glasgow and Edinburgh. He had been born in 1827, ten miles from London, at Upton Lodge, a Queen Anne house that later became a vicarage, in the small village of Upton in the county of Essex, now enmeshed in the dense urban area known as West Ham, E7. His father, a prosperous wine merchant in the City of London, was also a scientist with a major interest in optics. He had helped to improve the microscope by the development of the achromatic lens, and was a Fellow of the Royal Society (FRS).

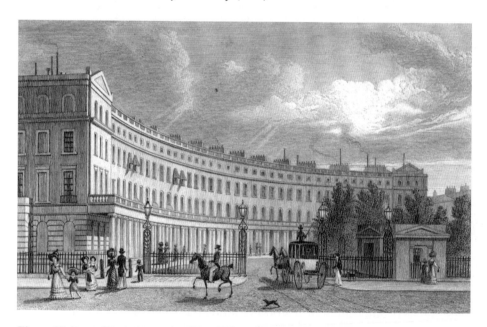

Figure 11 Part of Park Crescent, where Joseph Lister lived for thirty-four years, at Number 12. His house was almost 'round the corner' from Harley Street. From *London and Its Environs in the Nineteenth Century Illustrated by a Series of Views from Original Drawings by Thomas H. Shepherd* (London: James & Co., 1827).

The Listers were of pure Yorkshire stock, and despite spending twenty-four years of life in Scotland and having a Scottish wife, Joseph Lister (Figure 12) did not have any Scottish ancestry. After qualifying in medicine at University College Hospital and making a close study of physiology, he moved to Edinburgh to study under James Syme, Professor of Surgery in the University of Edinburgh. He became Syme's assistant, and in due course he married Syme's daughter. He remained a loyal admirer of Syme, but in 1861 he left Edinburgh to become

Professor of Surgery at the University of Glasgow. It was there that he pursued his studies into the nature of inflammation, and where he conceived the idea of 'sterilising' wounds with chemical solutions. For he had concluded, on the evidence of the brilliant work of Louis Pasteur in Paris, that suppuration in a wound was caused by 'particles' in the air and in the surroundings. These particles were in fact germs or, in more correct terminology, bacteria.

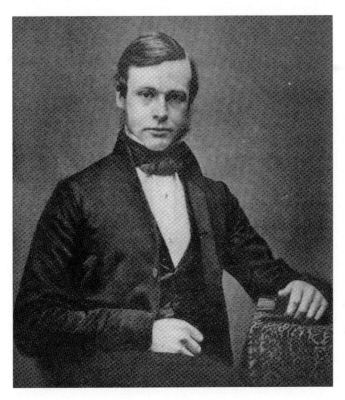

Figure 12 Joseph Lister as a young man. From *Joseph Lister: the friend of man by Hector Charles Cameron* (London: Heinemann, 1948). Reproduced with permission from the RSM Library.

A chemist rather than a doctor, Pasteur had studied such phenomena as putre-faction and fermentation, and had shown that these processes were caused by micro-organisms. He had indeed laid the foundation for the science of bacteri-ology (now microbiology), then in its infancy. He had shown that sheep and cows that had been vaccinated with attenuated anthrax bacteria were protected from the serious manifestations of anthrax even if they were then injected with virulent strains of the organism. Lister surmised, correctly, that if bacteria in the air and in a wound were killed, the wound would heal cleanly without suppu-ration – that is, 'by first intention'. After experimenting with various chemical solutions, he decided upon the use of carbolic acid to clear the wound of bacteria. There were some initial disappointments, but eventually his method proved successful in a substantial cohort of patients, and in 1867 he published in *The Lancet* the first of a series of papers in which he described the results of his technique. (Over a century and a half after the full acceptance of Lister's work, it is instructive again to read his original paper, which is reproduced in the Appendix to this book.) Operation wounds and wounds associated with fractures were sterilised with a 5 per cent watery solution of carbolic acid, as were the surgeon's hands and all the instruments used in an operation. Later, a weak solution of carbolic acid was sprayed into the air from a special machine as a fine mist, with the object of killing bacteria in the air.

As time went on, Lister's antiseptic methods had to be modified, partly because carbolic acid itself tended to cause some inflammation in a wound, and partly because inhalation of the mist of carbolic solution was unpleasant for those in the operation room, and possibly harmful. It turned out eventually that the only necessity was to sterilise (latterly by heat alone) all the instruments that were used in an operation, and so far as possible to sterilise the surgeon's and assistants' hands by very thorough washing in watery antiseptic solutions – and eventually by the provision of sterilised rubber gloves. Thus, Lister's antiseptic surgery was finally replaced by aseptic surgery, and modern surgery was born.

Meanwhile, in 1869, Lister had returned to Edinburgh as Professor of Surgery in succession to his father-in-law, James Syme. This was the period of his greatest success and satisfaction.

Lister in London

Eight years later, in 1877, Lister was invited to London to take the chair of surgery at King's College Hospital. He accepted this post, despite many personal reasons that might have kept him in Scotland, in order that his principles and discoveries might be more easily projected throughout the world from the bigger base of London. He had not appreciated, until he was back in London, that many of the surgeons there were reluctant to accept his ideas with the enthusiasm that was being shown elsewhere in Britain and in many centres overseas. He went through a difficult period; even some of his own colleagues at King's College Hospital were resentful, partly because he had insisted on bringing four assistants, trained in his technique, with him from Scotland. But this was not the only reason why surgeons in the metropolis were reluctant to accept Lister's ideas. There can be no doubt that a major factor was professional jealousy, which was (and still is) a real problem, not only in medicine but also in other walks of life. These colleagues of Lister saw that he was on to something big: they wished that they themselves could have been the ones to make the discoveries that he had made. In consequence, they came to belittle Lister's achievements, and almost subconsciously they hoped that Lister's work would prove in the end to be unsuccessful. But they could not hold out for ever. Before long it became clear to everyone that Lister was right and that his technique was attended by excellent results. It was being embraced enthusiastically by countless surgeons everywhere in the civilised world. The rebels had to join in, for fear of being left badly behind.

From then on, Lister was fêted as the enlightened innovator that he was. He received countless honours and was elected an honorary fellow of the surgical colleges of nearly every major country. He was made a baronet in 1883, and became a baron in 1897 – the first medical man to receive that honour. In 1902 he received the Order of Merit.

His last years were sad and lonely: his devoted wife had died in 1893, and there were no children. He gradually weakened in old age, and he died peacefully at Walmer on the Kent coast on 10 February 1912. At the public funeral service in Westminster Abbey there was sung an anthem composed by Handel, to words that are peculiarly appropriate to Lister's gentle nature:

> When the ear heard him, then it blessed him; and when the eye saw him, it gave witness of him; he delivered the poor that cried, the fatherless, and him that had none to help him. Kindness, meekness and comfort were on his tongue. If there was any virtue and if there was any praise, he thought on those things. His body is buried in peace, but his name liveth for evermore.

Celebrations of Joseph Lister's work

Joseph Lister gained huge acclaim in his lifetime and, unlike that of many famous people, his fame was long-lasting. Soon after his death a committee was formed, at the instigation of the Royal Society and the Royal College of Surgeons of England, with the object of commemorating 'the services of Lord Lister to science and the alleviation of human suffering'. The committee, after several meetings, suggested that there should be: in the first place, a tablet with medallion and inscription in Westminster Abbey; in the second place, a public monument in London; and in the third place, the establishment of an international memorial fund for the advancement of surgery, from which grants in aid of research, or awards in recognition of distinguished contributions to surgical science, should be made, irrespective of nationality.

These objectives were duly achieved. In the north transept of Westminster Abbey a marble medallion of Lister's bust was placed near to those of the great scientists Darwin, Stokes, Anderson and Watt. An appeal was launched after a meeting at the Mansion House in London, which met with responses from all over the world, a total of £12,000 being received – a large sum at the time.

The public memorial to Lord Lister was unveiled on 13 March 1924. It stands in the middle of the road at the northern end of Portland Place. The base and pedestal are of grey Aberdeen granite, and on the summit is a large bust in bronze of Lord Lister, with a wreath in front enclosing the first letter of his name. Below are life-size figures of a woman, representing humanity, and a child holding a garland. One of the woman's hands rests on the child's shoulder, and with the other she points upwards to the bust. On one side of the pedestal is the word

'Surgery', with a device below incorporating the Aesculapian rod and the two-headed serpent, and on the other side the word 'Science', and below this a flaming torch. On the back of the pedestal are Lister's dates, 1827–1912. The bronze work on the memorial was carried out by Sir Thomas Brock, RA (1847–1922).

A memorial was also erected in 1924 in a small garden in Kelvingrove Park, Glasgow, below the tower of Glasgow University. It is a life-size statue by H. D. Parkin of Lord Lister, seated. It commemorates Lister's work during the period in which he was Professor of Surgery in Glasgow.

There have been many subsequent celebrations of Lister's life and work, most notably those staged in April 1927 to mark the centenary of his birth. The huge scale of those celebrations was staggering, even when it is remembered that Lister had then been dead for less than fifteen years, and that there were many people still alive who had known him, or even worked with him. Such widespread acclamation is rare indeed, and probably unprecedented.

The events began at Buckingham Palace in London, where delegates were honoured by the presence of King George V. A week-long programme of tributes to Lister followed, with celebrations at the Royal Society of Medicine in Wimpole Street; at Lister's birthplace, at Upton in Essex; in Glasgow; at King's College Hospital in London; and at the British Medical Association's house in London, where a reception was given by the Prime Minister.

The highlight of the celebrations in London was the reception at Buckingham Palace, at which was assembled a large gathering of scientists, academics, surgeons, physicians and others, with many delegates from overseas as well as from what were then the dominions of Australia, Canada, India, New Zealand and South Africa. An address was presented to the King by Sir Ernest Rutherford, President of the Royal Society, in which the work of Lister was described as having done more for the saving of human life and the prevention and relief of suffering than the scientific activity of any other man. Brilliant qualities of investigation had been necessary in applying the discoveries of Pasteur to the problems of wound infection.

The King in reply said:

> I thank you for the address which you have presented. It is with pleasure that I receive the delegates who are present here today, and so take part in the Centenary commemoration of Lord Lister's birth. Any country might be proud to claim Lord Lister as its citizen; and I and my people heartily welcome the representatives of medical and surgical science, both from the Overseas Dominions and from all parts of the civilised world who have come to join us in honouring his memory. You have truly said that Lister ranks among the greatest benefactors to mankind. Of all the many changes in the last 100 years none is more striking than the revolution in thought concerning surgery. It is hard now to realise the dread and apprehension with

which formerly even a minor surgical operation was regarded. This change in our ideas is due partly to the discovery of anaesthetics but perhaps even more to Lister's work. Lister removed the horror of sepsis from surgical operations, and for this he is rightly described as the father of modern surgery. The principles discovered and laid down by him are today being worked out by his successors and are still fruitful of new applications.... It is my earnest desire and hope that the Lister Centenary Celebrations may be in every way successful, and that this gathering of men of science from every quarter of the globe may conduce to foster and to strengthen the cooperation of all nations in the accumulation of scientific knowledge for the common benefit of the human race.

Among the commemorative papers presented during a notable week of celebrations at the Royal Society of Medicine in April 1927 was an address by Sir St-Clair Thomson, then a distinguished laryngologist, who had served as one of Lister's house surgeons at King's College Hospital in 1883. The following extracts from his address give an insight into the medical atmosphere of the time, and of the veneration with which Lister was regarded by his juniors:

During the siege of Paris (1870–71) Nelaton, in despair at the sight of the death of almost every patient after operation, declared that he who should conquer purulent infection would deserve a statue made of gold. This passage occurs in *The Life of Pasteur*. One hundred years ago tomorrow, on April 5th, 1827, Joseph Lister was born; the man through whose work surgical purulent infection was conquered for all humanity and for all time. There is a ... bust of him in Portland Place, but the statue of gold has not yet been erected, although wound infection was conquered in Lister's own lifetime. Lister achieved more for mankind than all the surgeons from the beginning of history. Before his coming the results of surgical wounds were hardly better than in the dark ages, and yet he lived to see his work and teaching result in the saving of more lives than all the military heroes of all the ages have destroyed.

Lister, a simple and a noble man, could never have understood the spirit of the poet who exclaimed: 'Let fame which all hunt after be written on our tombs.' If, indeed, Lister ever had hankered after posthumous fame, it would probably have been the words of Byron he would have quoted: 'My epitaph shall be my name alone.'

When Lister came to London bacteriology as a science was non-existent: the connection of fermentation and putrefaction with the healing of wounds was unknown or scouted, or even ridiculed: if a wound healed by 'first intention' it was looked on as an exception, and the rule was that suppuration was Nature's usual process of repair, and that pus might even be, as it was termed in those days, 'laudable'....

[Lister's] first plunge in the lecture theatre at King's College was chilly, but it was at the [King's College] Hospital that Lister encountered his full sea of trouble. He had stipulated that he should be allowed to bring with him from Edinburgh four assistants already trained in his methods, and attached solely to his service. This was a cause of offence, because in those days operations were so few that one house surgeon, and one operating theatre, were sufficient for all the surgeons on the staff....

The peace-loving Quaker spirit of Lister was also much distressed by the opposition that he met with at the hospital from the nursing sisters of St John. At that date the hospital authorities farmed out, so to speak, their nursing to an Anglican community much given to ritual, frigid rules, repressive formality, and petty restrictions. In the days of Sir William Fergusson [Lister's predecessor] the teaching was entirely in the wards; he passed from bed to bed, followed by a sister with a towel and a basin of water, in which he dipped his hands after examining a patient. Lister upset the pious sisters by copious ablutions and the purification of many pairs of hands before a patient was touched, and many of his patients were carried or wheeled into the theatre as subjects for clinical lectures. These sisters of St John were opposed to Lister and all his ways, and dealt him those pious and smiling stabs in which women, and particularly good women, are so skilful. Patient, courteous, self-controlled, Lister exhibited no resentment, never retaliated, and only showed how he felt it by the little gasping sigh we all learned to know and to respect as his only sign of sorrow or anger....

But if students and London surgeons were apathetic over the revolution in surgery being wrought in their very midst, it was not so with the foreigners. When I was house surgeon with Lister, forty-four years ago, there was in the entrance hall of the old hospital a painted notice board forbidding smoking in English, French and German. It read thus:

> Smoking is forbidden.
> Il est defendu de fumer.
> Das Rauchen ist verboten.

In 1883 foreigners poured into King's College Hospital, from the ends of the earth, crowded the entrance hall, and there, while waiting for the master, they would make the air thick with tobacco smoke. In later years, when Lister's evangel had gone forth over all the earth, and he was neglected by both students and visitors, many must have wondered at the need of this polyglot announcement. It survived as a memento of the few early years in London when the prophet was still without honour in his own country, but was attracting from overseas the seekers after truth. Already in 1875, two years before coming to London, Lister, during a prolonged tour in Germany, was received everywhere with enthusiasm. In the words of *The Lancet*, 'the progress of Professor Lister has assumed the character of a triumphal march.' In 1879 Lister's appearances at the International Congress of Medicine at Amsterdam were greeted with 'an enthusiasm which knew no bounds.'

At the next International Congress in London in 1881 foreign surgeons must have marvelled amongst themselves when they heard British surgeons still attempting to cast doubts on his principles or belittle his results. But let us, in parenthesis, project our attention forward to the following International Congress in London. It was in 1913. Lister had died in the previous year, but the light of his good work was shining before all men. As is well known, congresses and such like events are often commemorated by the issue of a medal. The medal of 1881, when Lister's work was slighted and belittled by his own countrymen, bore the features of Queen Victoria. But in 1913 it was felt in Britain that the one effigy worthy of being stamped on the medal of the International Congress in London was the head of Joseph Lister.

My audience will hardly believe me when I tell them that in my student days the surgeons of one of the largest teaching hospitals – a Fellow of the Royal Society, and a president of the Royal College of Surgeons – frequently raised an appreciative laugh by telling any one who came into his operating theatre to shut the door quickly, 'in case one of Mr Lister's microbes should come in.'...

In those early years of Lister's advent a little personal recollection will illustrate how slowly his gospel spread, yet how courageously confident the master was of his mission. One day, in 1883, after he had been six years in London, I was standing beside him on the steps of the hospital, waiting (as is the way with deferential house surgeons) for his carriage to pull up. We had been discussing the attack made on him for having the temerity to open a healthy knee joint. He began by quietly remarking that the day must come when the profession would accept the principles of his methods; 'and', he added warmly, 'if the profession does not recognise them, the public will learn of them, and the law will insist on them.' Then, placing his hand on my shoulder, he added pathetically, 'Thomson, I do not expect to live to see that day, but you may.'

Shortly afterwards I went abroad and spent some years on the Continent. To state that I had been Lister's house surgeon served as a *laissez-passer* to make me welcome in any foreign hospital I visited. Everywhere I found Listerian principles had been embraced and his methods pursued with brilliant success. When I settled again in London in 1893 I found the whole surgical atmosphere had changed during my ten years' absence. Younger surgeons, more open to conviction and less wedded to old routine, had come along, and late converts concealed their overdue repentance by rapturously embracing asepsis, and vaunting its superiority over the 'antiseptic' system, as it was still called. Soon after my return, in 1897, the year of Queen Victoria's second jubilee, Lister was made a peer on New Year's Day, his peerage having been the first ever conferred upon a surgeon. In a picture of his coat-of-arms you will notice that the serpent of Aesculapius, for the first time in history, appears in the quarterings of a peer of the realm....

What was the personality of this master of surgery? He was tall, upright, well knit, stoutly built, deep-chested; his bearing was dignified, and his manner always serious, restrained, courteous, and considerate. He had a profusion of thick iron-grey hair, worn somewhat long, as had been the fashion in his youth. Except for small side-whiskers, he was clean shaven. I never saw him in any other pattern of collar or necktie than those seen in all his portraits; a black silk bow tie and an upright collar with the peaks turned down over it. His costume never varied; he always wore a frock coat made of the shiny black material called broadcloth, and nowadays only seen on undertakers and country hotel waiters.... He commanded not only veneration, respect and admiration, but a feeling of complete trust and devotion which could only be explained by the nobility and sincerity of his character....

Lister was born a Quaker, but lived most of his life and died a member of the Church of England. He was blessed with a loving and devoted wife. She was the daughter of Professor Syme, whom he had served as house surgeon in Edinburgh, and she appeared to have no thought or interest beyond her husband. She not only loved and shielded him in every way, but entered intelligently into all his work and researches; helped him in his studies; worked in his laboratory; wrote his letters; and always when I arrived at his house in the early morning to go with him to a private operation I would find Mrs Lister preparing and checking off his instruments. In their pleasures as in their work they were united. They were inseparable companions on all his holidays, and in the numerous Continental trips he loved to make. It was while on one of these in Italy that his wife died, after a brief illness, in 1893. They had no children, and after her death Lister was a lonely man.

On 5 April 1927 there were further commemorations of Joseph Lister's birth at Upton House, his birthplace in the village of Upton in Essex, then largely invaded by the suburban sprawl of London in the district of West Ham. The address was given by Sir Humphrey Rolleston, physician to St George's Hospital, of 55 Upper Brook Street, central London – then equal to Harley Street as a prestigious address from which to practise medicine.

After giving a brief outline of Lister's background and career, Sir Humphrey described the worldwide transformation of surgery that was brought about by his work on 'antiseptic surgery'. He said:

> The history of surgery has indeed been divided into two periods, that before and that after Lister's methods became adopted. Before his discovery, as few operations as possible were done, because of the risk that they would be followed by erysipelas, blood poisoning, pyaemia, hospital gangrene, tetanus, and death. Abdominal operations such as are so constantly done now for appendicitis were practically unknown; to open a large abscess was almost certainly to sign the patient's death warrant. Hospitals indeed were spoken of as 'houses of death.'

Sir Humphrey concluded by recalling that:

> ... like Pasteur, and more fortunate than many reformers and pioneers, Lister lived to see his work bear fruit exceedingly, and died full of years and loaded with honours from all countries; but it is as the greatest material benefactor of the human race, who made surgery safe, and thereby did more than any other man to prevent suffering and save life, that we regard him with deep gratitude and thankfulness.

Other centenary celebrations were held in Glasgow, where, at a civic luncheon, an address was given by Sir John Bland-Sutton, former President of the Royal College of Surgeons of England. After summarising Lister's career and work, he emphasised how, in consequence of Lister's discoveries, surgery had been utterly transformed:

> In the face of opposition, Lister pursued his course apparently unruffled. The younger surgeons – enthusiastic converts – adopted his principles and gradually introduced the methods of the bacteriological laboratory, sterilisation by heat. This ultimately became the Cult of Asepsis. Indeed, heat is the most perfect antiseptic known. Odoriferous carbolic acid persists as a memory. Since 1900 operative surgery has advanced with such strides that textbooks of surgery have become like railway time-tables, useful only for a season. Surgical methods change monthly. Operating theatres, which resembled shambles in 1860, are replaced by rooms of spotless purity containing scintillating metal furniture and ingenious electric lights.

> All concerned in the operation are clothed from nose-tip to toe-tip in sterilised linen garments, and their hands [are] covered with sterilised rubber gloves. The patient is in a sleep as deep as that of Adam in Eden; and the theatrical silence is only broken by the rhythmical breathing of the patient or an occasional utterance from a nervous operator. Modern surgery is wonderful. I was trained in the old school and lived to revel in the wonders of the new.

In the afternoon delegates visited Kelvingrove Park in Glasgow and laid wreaths at the foot of the Lister monument.

At King's College Hospital itself, where Lister spent the last sixteen years of his active professional life, celebrations had been arranged by the Listerian Society, under the chairmanship of the Society's President, Mr Arthur Cheatle. The address was given by Sir William Watson Cheyne, who had been Joseph Lister's house surgeon in Edinburgh and had come to King's College Hospital with him to act as his house surgeon there. Sir William reminded the audience that it was during the time that Lister spent at King's College Hospital that he completed the simplification of his method of treating wounds. Sir William gave examples of Lister's extreme conscientiousness and his complete freedom from affectation:

> Apart from this conscientiousness Lister was full of sympathy for sufferers, and was always ready to do what he could to relieve suffering and to help those in need. One has only to look at his portraits to see these characteristics beautifully depicted.

After Cheyne's address, Sir Lenthal Cheatle joined in welcoming many old friends at the large gathering, including Mr Hamilton Russell, who had travelled from Melbourne in Australia. Sir Lenthal regarded Lister as in every way the greatest man he had ever met. His devotion to his work and his courtesy caused all who had dealings with him to revere him. Russell, who had worked with Lister in his youth before he had emigrated to Australia, recalled Lister's immense skill in dressing wounds at the bedside. 'Every action in Lister's daily life showed that he loved his fellow men; he had the philanthropic temperament, and would point out that when the patient was a child [the doctor's] responsibilities were increased'.

A fitting finale to this intense week of celebrations was a reception given by the Prime Minister, Mr Stanley Baldwin, in the great hall of the British Medical Association's building in London, where the chair was taken by Sir Ernest Rutherford, President of the Royal Society. Delegates from no less than twenty-two foreign countries and sixty-two British institutions were received by the Prime Minister. Mr Baldwin said that the boundaries of all the nations were broken down in that hall. He recalled the words of a great American Ambassador who, at a dinner of the Royal Society, had said: 'My Lord [Lister], it is not a profession, it is not a nation, it is humanity itself which, with uncovered head, salutes you.'

Today's appraisal of Lister's work

Over a century and a half after Lister first described his method of 'antiseptic surgery', he is still applauded as the first to recognise the role of air-born 'particles' (bacteria) in the causation of wound infection, and to tell the world how this calamitous complication of surgical operations could be prevented.

At the celebrations of the centenary of his birth described above, there were many people still alive who had known him personally, and they relished the opportunity to refresh their memories of him. Today, with the passage of time, as often happens, there is a tendency to take our present blessings for granted, and to forget how it all came about. It would be wrong, however, to suggest that Lister has been wholly forgotten. But if further celebrations were proposed in the future, it is unlikely that there would be an enthusiastic response. Time does indeed kill fame. There is a present tendency to neglect the past and to think more about current problems. Ironically, these now include the emergence of virulent and hardy bacteria, resistant to most antibiotics, that are again causing devastating infection of operation wounds – the very complication that Lister went so far to eliminate – though fortunately not at present on the scale of the pre-Listerian period.

There is also the problem of rival heroes competing for recognition and fame: pioneers such as Wilhelm Conrad Roentgen (1845–1923), discoverer of X-rays; Alexander Fleming (1881–1955), the Scottish microbiologist who in 1928 discovered penicillin at St Mary's Hospital in London; the Oxford Professors Howard Florey (1898–1968) and Ernst Chain (1906–79), who developed penicillin for clinical use; and Albert Sabin (1906–93), who virtually rid the Western world of poliomyelitis (infantile paralysis), that terrible paralysing disease that took thousands of lives and left countless others (including the American President Franklin D. Roosevelt) disabled.

Fleming received huge acclaim at the time of his death, but in retrospect he has to forfeit some of the fame that he might have achieved, because of two misjudgements. First, having observed that colonies of bacteria on a culture plate left out while he took a holiday had been eliminated (lysed) by a mould that had settled on the plate, he initially regarded this as just an interesting observation and threw the culture plate into the waste bin. It was only through the intervention of his assistant, Merlin Pryce, later Professor of Pathology at St Mary's Hospital, that the priceless plate was retrieved. 'Hang on,' Pryce exclaimed, 'there could be something important here. Don't throw the plate away.' Secondly, Fleming failed to follow up the potential of his discovery for clinical use; it was left to Chain and Florey of Oxford, with their brilliant chemist assistant Norman Keatley, to do this in the early 1940s, in the teeth of oppressive restrictions imposed by the Second World War. Fleming, Chain and Florey shared the 1945 Nobel Prize for Physiology or Medicine.

Albert Sabin seems not to have achieved the acclaim that he deserved, bearing in mind that he prevented untold thousands of deaths from poliomyelitis.

Lister happened to be the man on the spot at the right time: the time when Louis Pasteur, the brilliant French chemist, had just shown that putrefaction and fermentation were caused by living micro-organisms. The time was ripe for someone to prove that micro-organisms were also the cause of wound infection and suppuration, and that if they were kept out of the wound, or killed, such complications would not occur. Had Lister not been on the scene, these facts would certainly have been discovered by another observer, probably within quite a short time, for the evidence was already there.

Indeed, some twenty years before Lister's reports, Ignaz Philipp Semmelweiss (1818–65), a Hungarian obstetrician then (1847) working in Vienna, had noticed a relationship between the frequent passage of medical students from the anatomy dissecting room to the obstetric wards, and puerperal fever, horrendously common at that time and a major cause of death in women after childbirth. He suspected that some kind of contaminant brought in with the students might be the cause. After he had enforced rules that the obstetric ward should be cleaned regularly with calcium chloride, and that the staff should wash their hands very carefully before attending to patients, the death rate from puerperal sepsis in his wards fell dramatically. His observations were reported to the Vienna Medical Society in 1847 but, like Lister in 1867, he was ridiculed by many of his colleagues.

In America, too, Oliver Wendell Holmes (1841–1935), an obstetrician who also advocated extreme cleanliness in the obstetric wards on the grounds that puerperal fever was contagious and might be introduced on the attendant's hands, suffered similar ridicule from his colleagues. In Italy, Enrico Bottini (1835–1903) had experimented with the use of carbolic acid as a disinfectant of operation wounds at about the same time that Lister was working with carbolic acid in Glasgow.

It is clear that people were beginning to get an inkling of the truth. But it was left to Joseph Lister to put all this together and to publish his results in 1867. It so happened that the person who was able to achieve this was a man of great personal charm, with a deep compassion for suffering mankind. This undoubtedly endeared him to those who came into contact with him, and enhanced his reputation among the wider public and the profession, who were increasingly ready to accept his teaching.

Chapter 5

The generation after Lister

Surgeons in practice after the period of Lister's innovations had the great advantage that they could expect their operation wounds to heal cleanly, without the dreaded complications of infection and suppuration. Their scope for surgery was enormously widened, and the number of operations that were undertaken greatly increased. There was a general awareness among doctors of the important part that micro-organisms (bacteria) played not only in relation to skin wounds but also in medical problems such as pneumonia and the common fevers. Seeing the increased safety of surgery, many more doctors presented themselves for training in the specialty, in which the perspective was radically altered.

Sir Rickman Godlee

One surgeon who achieved fame from his close association with Lister was Rickman John Godlee (1849–1925). Godlee's mother was Joseph Lister's sister, so Godlee was Lister's nephew. His father was of a dedicated Quaker family and Rickman Godlee followed the Quaker way of life, studying botany and nature in the countryside as a boy. He qualified in medicine in 1872, from University College Hospital in London, gaining a gold medal in surgery. He then went to Edinburgh, where Lister's work was proceeding apace, and where its importance was perhaps more fully recognised than it was in London at the time. He worked there as Lister's assistant and acquired a full knowledge of the principles and practice of 'antiseptic surgery'. Returning then to London, he was appointed as assistant surgeon to University College Hospital and demonstrator of anatomy at the medical school there. He had the advantage of being a first-class draughtsman, some of whose illustrations were used in textbooks of anatomy.

When Lister himself came to London in 1877 as Professor of Surgery, Godlee again became his regular assistant. He had a lucrative practice of his own at 19 Wimpole Street, and he achieved some distinction in medical circles when he removed a glioma (brain tumour) in a patient aged twenty-five after its precise location in the brain had been defined by Dr Hughes Bennett, a leading neurologist of the day. Such operations had seldom been attempted before, and the case sparked much debate, in the national press as well as among doctors, as to whether it was ethically acceptable to operate upon the human brain. Some contended that such an operation was tantamount to vivisection. Medical opinion, however, was that the case demonstrated the feasibility of surgical removal of cerebral tumours, and that this was an important landmark.

In 1884 Godlee was appointed as surgeon to the Brompton Hospital, the well known centre in London for the treatment of respiratory diseases. He became proficient in operating upon the lungs, and with his colleague Sir James Kingston Fowler he wrote a book, *Diseases of the Lungs*, which proved to be a timely addition to the medical literature of the time.

After a long association with the Royal College of Surgeons of England, Godlee was elected its President in 1911, and he was knighted in 1914, on the termination of his three-year period of office. In his retirement at Coombe End Farm on Whitchurch Hill, overlooking the Thames in Oxfordshire, he wrote a biography of Lord Lister, in which the development of antiseptic surgery was recalled in detail.

Sir Frederick Treves

Among the most famous of the second, or post-Lister, generation of surgeons in the Harley Street area was Sir Frederick Treves, Bart (1853–1923), who lived and practised at 6 Wimpole Street, in a house that still stands. Treves was a skilful abdominal surgeon who was sometime Professor of Surgery at London University and surgeon to the London Hospital, where he had received his medical training. He achieved instant fame when he was called upon to operate upon King Edward VII for acute appendicitis. Edward had succeeded to the throne after the death of his mother, Queen Victoria, on 22 January 1901, and his coronation was imminent when this surgical emergency arose. The situation was such that the coronation had to be postponed. After the diseased appendix had been removed successfully by Treves, the delayed coronation took place on 9 August 1901. It is clear that, in all probability, the operation saved the life of King Edward VII: had it not been for the advancement of surgery consequent upon the work of Lister, there is a strong possibility that he might have died from the appendicular infection.

Treves was a prolific author, writing or contributing to several surgical textbooks. He made a detailed study of the anatomy of the abdominal organs, and wrote authoritatively on acute appendicitis, then known as perityphlitis. His practice flourished after the well publicised operation upon the King, so that he was able to retire at the age of fifty, to indulge in world travel, of which he wrote entertaining accounts. His *Elephant Man and Other Reminiscences* (1823) affords interesting reading.

After the royal appendicectomy it became fashionable, among a certain type of patient, to seek to have the appendix removed electively. No doubt a great many appendices were removed unnecessarily during this period.

Sir Victor Horsley

Sir Victor Horsley (1857–1916) was another surgeon fortunate enough to reach his prime after Lister's introduction of antiseptic surgery. After his medical training at University College Hospital, where he gained a gold medal in the examination in surgery, he was quickly appointed as assistant surgeon, and later as full surgeon, to that hospital. He was also appointed as surgeon to the National Hospital in Queen Square, London, the leading institute for the study and practice of neurology and neurosurgery.

Successful though he was as a general surgeon, it was soon apparent that Horsley's interests lay predominantly in scientific research, with particular reference to the anatomy and physiology of the nervous system; and in the development of techniques of neurosurgery, a branch of surgery in which he was a pioneer. Brain surgery and the surgery of the spinal cord indeed formed a field that had hardly been explored at all: before the work of Lister, it would have been foolhardy to entertain any thought of exposing the brain or the nerve tissues.

Horsley was one of the first surgeons to carry out successfully an operation for the removal of a brain tumour. He also pioneered the removal of brain substance for the relief of traumatic epilepsy. In 1887 he undertook for the first time the operation of laminectomy (exposure of the spinal cord) for removal of a spinal tumour. So prominent had his work become that he was received with great acclaim when he attended the International Medical Congress in Berlin in 1890. He ventured into almost every aspect of brain and spinal cord surgery, at a time when localisation of brain lesions was still far from refined.

Horsley also studied the surgery of the thyroid gland, paving the way for the use of thyroxin in the treatment of thyroid deficiency. He died while at the height of his powers, allegedly from sunstroke while on military service in Mesopotamia in 1916.

Sir George Frederick Still

Sir George Frederick Still (1868–1941) was from a slightly later generation. Like Joseph Lister three decades previously, he became a consultant surgeon at King's College Hospital in London. He lived and practised privately at 28 Queen Anne Street, which intersects Harley Street. Trained at Cambridge and Guy's Hospital, he worked at the Great Ormond Street Hospital for Sick Children before becoming Professor of the Diseases of Children at King's College Hospital. In his later years he was physician to Princess Elizabeth, later to become Queen Elizabeth II, and her sister Princess Margaret. He is remembered today for his paper entitled 'On a form of chronic joint disease in children', describing what is often referred to now as Still's disease.

Sir William Arbuthnot Lane

Another famous personality of this post-Listerian period, but still in the heyday of Harley Street practice, was Sir William Arbuthnot Lane (1856–1943). Like Frederick Still, Lane qualified at Guy's Hospital. He established a successful private practice at 21 Cavendish Square, a prestigious address where Lord Asquith was his neighbour. Though always a general surgeon, Lane tended towards the practice of bone surgery. He devised many surgical instruments that are still used in bone and joint surgery today, as well as others used in abdominal surgery.

To minimise the risk of infection of the wound after operations (still feared even after Lister's work had been accepted worldwide), Lane advocated a system of 'no-touch' surgery, in which the 'business end' of the surgical instruments – that is, the part that entered the wound – never came into contact with the surgeon's or assistants' hands, which might, he thought, be contaminated with germs, through carelessness or accident. The hands themselves, or anything that had been touched by the hands, were never allowed to enter the wound, again on the grounds that the fingers were potentially contaminated – as indeed they probably often were at the time. Suture needles had to be held in forceps and the sutures themselves were guided through the needle's eye with forceps, not with the fingers. Lane's 'no touch' technique, seemingly difficult to master but not so in practice, was adopted by many other surgeons and, indeed, is still used by some; but it has proved rather too demanding for today's surgeons, who dislike being deprived of the facility of handling tissues, metalwork and prostheses inside the wound, and who regard this 'fiddling' technique as unnecessary in these days of powerful antibiotics. It has to be said, however, that it served a useful service in its time and must have been responsible for preventing scores of disastrous infections in surgical wounds, and thus for saving many lives.

Lane was a pioneer of the internal fixation of fractured bones, especially by metal plates and screws. But his principles and techniques were ahead of advances in metallurgy. His plating operations were often successful, but the plates and screws, made from ordinary carbon steel, reacted with the tissues and eventually corroded. If removed months or years later, the plates were partly corroded away and the screws might be so attenuated that they could simply be lifted out. The metal was rusty and the surrounding tissues were stained brown with iron oxide. Despite this late failure of the metal, the plates had usually served their purpose and promoted healing of the fracture long before corrosion became significant. It was some years after Lane's time that stainless steels and other metals that were resistant to corrosion in the body were introduced.

Aside from his work on bones and joints, Lane's main interest was in abdominal surgery. His superb operative skill led him into some controversy with his colleagues. For he advocated to excess the major operation of colectomy (excision of part of the colon) in the belief that it harboured organisms that could reach the blood stream and cause harm elsewhere in the body. He believed that 'intestinal stasis' was the cause of much ill-health, and that it could best be cured by colectomy. This was a dubious concept in any case, and a foolhardy one when the magnitude of the operation of colectomy is borne in mind. Lane's views were strongly contested by many abdominal surgeons who, while respecting his surgical skill, took him to task at a meeting at the Royal Society of Medicine in 1922. He was not dissuaded, however, and continued to practise the operation, in the opinion of most surgeons greatly hazarding the health of his patients.

The beginnings of orthopaedic surgery

Orthopaedic surgery was a specialty that arrived late on the Harley Street scene. The word 'orthopaedic' had been coined in France by Nicolas Andry (1658–1742) in a book on the prevention and treatment of childhood deformities published in 1741. It is derived from the Greek words *orthos* (straight) and *pais* or *paedion* (child) and, as these words imply, the specialty was initially concerned almost entirely with the correction, or attempted correction, of childhood deformities, often club foot or spinal curvature. In the absence of the antiseptic principles put forward by Lister in 1867, the early orthopaedic surgeons had to avoid operating upon bones or joints, on account of the almost universal complication of disastrous infection, which, even if it did not kill the patient, certainly nullified the object of the operation.

These so-called orthopaedic surgeons were therefore widely despised, especially by the general surgeons, who could at least undertake certain 'cutting' operations, even though many of them were destructive, in the form of amputations. In their view, orthopaedic surgeons were merely 'mechanicians', concerned only with the application of external splints or 'instruments'. A well known orthopaedic surgeon of the period, who joined the staff of the Royal National Orthopaedic Hospital in London, described how, as a student soon to qualify in medicine, he was told that 'orthopaedic surgery is dead'; his teachers tried to dissuade him from taking up orthopaedic surgery as a career. This strong antipathy to orthopaedic surgery was shared by much of the medical press. The editor of a leading medical journal, writing in 1872 on the subject of an orthopaedic hospital of which the domestic affairs had attracted unwanted prominence, ranted: 'Cut it down; why cumbereth it the ground? There is not … the shadow of a pretence for saying that it is required to meet a public want.'

Muirhead Little

In fact, there was a place for special hospitals, including orthopaedic hospitals. As Muirhead Little (1854–1935) pointed out, nearly all progress in the surgery of the eye, and in the surgery of the ear, nose and throat, was attributable to specialists working in dedicated institutions – notably the Moorfields Eye Hospital and the Hospital for Diseases of the Throat. As it turned out, Muirhead Little himself, whose father was remembered for his description of a form of infantile spastic paralysis that became known as Little's disease, had a successful career in orthopaedic surgery. He was largely instrumental in the foundation in 1918 of the British Orthopaedic Association, of which he was the first President. His surgical career was spent almost entirely at the Royal National Orthopaedic Hospital in Great Portland Street, where he was senior surgeon for many years. He lived and practised privately in Seymour Street, a short distance from Harley Street.

Struggle for recognition

Orthopaedic surgeons did have a long struggle to gain recognition of their work and potential, even after they had thrown off the adverse publicity that arose from their former status as 'mechanicians' dependent upon cumbersome appliances for the correction of deformity. Their early experience of 'cutting' surgery was almost confined to the simple operation of tenotomy (division of contracted tendons close under the skin); any open operation on a bone or joint was so hazardous that, before Lister's time, it had to be avoided. Even after the general adoption of safer surgery derived from the work of Lister, they failed at first to gain recognition from the general surgeons, who continued to guard their position as the sole purveyors of surgery. General surgeons denied orthopaedists the privilege of treating fractures, now considered an important part of an orthopaedic surgeon's role. So insistent were they upon their rights that the major teaching hospitals were slow to appoint orthopaedic surgeons to their staff. Orthopaedic work was therefore by necessity carried out at specialist orthopaedic hospitals.

In London the main such hospital was the Royal National Orthopaedic Hospital, founded in 1907 through the amalgamation of two small existing hospitals, the Royal Orthopaedic Hospital and the National Orthopaedic Hospital. A third hospital, the City Orthopaedic Hospital, was incorporated later. The earliest orthopaedic appointments to the staffs of London teaching hospitals were not made before about 1908, and at the most conservative hospitals, such as St Mary's in Paddington, the 1930s had dawned before any orthopaedic surgeon was appointed.

Sir Robert Jones

It was in the First World War that the obstructions faced by orthopaedic surgeons were finally broken, through the work of one of the most famous orthopaedic surgeons of all time, Sir Robert Jones (1858–1933). Robert Jones began his career in Liverpool, where his uncle, Hugh Owen Thomas – descended from a family line of bone-setters but himself a qualified doctor – had gained a wide reputation for the management of limb injuries and diseases of joints. Robert Jones trained as an orthopaedic surgeon and during the First World War, already highly esteemed, he was appointed as Inspector of Military Orthopaedics. This was a key position and Jones, a fine organiser, made the most of it. He established a train of special hospitals for the treatment of soldiers who had sustained injuries to the limbs and spine, the most notable of which were the Military Orthopaedic Hospital at Shepherd's Bush, London, and the Alder Hey Hospital in Liverpool. With the help of American orthopaedic colleagues who came over in the war to help British surgeons, he trained a whole team, who were then sent out to the battle zones to man their individual units. His insistence on the use of the Thomas's knee splint (the invention of his uncle) saved the lives of hundreds of soldiers with gunshot wounds and fractures of the thigh.

Jones was knighted in 1917 for his services to medicine, and was appointed a baronet in 1926. After the war he was appointed as the first consulting orthopaedic surgeon to St Thomas's Hospital, with Rowley Bristow, of 102 Harley Street, as his deputy. He led an incredibly busy life, with consultant work not only in Liverpool but also in London, where at first he practised at 9 Cavendish Square, adjacent to Harley Street. Later he moved to the fashionable Mayfair district of central London, to consult at 116 Park Street, near Grosvenor Square. He took a prominent part in the foundation of the British Orthopaedic Association in 1918 and served as its second President for five years, from 1921 to 1925. He was assisted in his work for the Association by Harry Platt (later Sir Harry), of Manchester, the only orthopaedic surgeon to have lived to be a hundred years old, from 1886 to 1986.

Without doubt, Sir Robert Jones was the most respected and, indeed, the best-loved orthopaedic surgeon of all time. He retained his magnetic charm unspoilt, regardless of his worldwide fame. He was revered in America and on the Continent of Europe, being elected as honorary fellow of the orthopaedic associations of all the major European countries; and he received almost countless other honours.

Sir Thomas Fairbank

Another pioneer of orthopaedic surgery was Sir Thomas Fairbank (1876–1961). Trained in medicine at the Charing Cross Hospital, after having already obtained a qualification in dental surgery, he began his career at the Hospital for Sick Children in Great Ormond Street, London, where he was later to serve as consultant orthopaedic surgeon for the greater part of his career. But the South African War intervened, and he served there as surgeon in the Royal Army Medical Corps until the war ended. In 1908 he was appointed as consultant orthopaedic surgeon at the Charing Cross Hospital – the first ever orthopaedic surgeon to be appointed at a London teaching hospital. He was again in uniform during the First World War, when he served on the western front in France and later in Salonika.

A junior colleague with whom he had worked at the Charing Cross Hospital later recalled how delighted he was when Fairbank unexpectedly turned up to tend to wounded soldiers at a regimental aid post in the battle area, in the cellar of a French chateau that had been commandeered as a makeshift hospital:

> I was in a devil of a fix. The room was full of wounded. Suddenly the
> field ambulance bearers burst in, and who should be in charge but

Captain Fairbank? Never was a young regimental medical officer more relieved and pleased; for Fairbank was his old teacher and revered chief. I remember the care he took in applying the Thomas's splint and dressing the wound; how quiet he was and cheerful when we were all depressed. It was a night of heavy shelling around our post, but 'Tommy F.' was so calm, and as brave as a lion.

Later, in Salonika, Fairbank the experienced surgeon was detailed to take the post of transport officer in charge of mules – a hilarious situation for the group of medical officers whom he was to join: a senior surgeon in charge of mules. Such were the vagaries of life in the services. But in due course right prevailed, and Fairbank took on his true role as senior surgeon.

Back in London after the war, Fairbank was appointed as the first consultant orthopaedic surgeon to King's College Hospital, where he established the first daily outpatient fracture clinic in London, the second in the whole of England. He served as consultant to many other hospitals, as well as the Hospital for Sick Children in Great Ormond Street. These included the world-famous Lord Mayor Treloar Orthopaedic Hospital at Alton in Hampshire, now sadly extinct.

Fairbank was so widely respected in his lifetime that for his eightieth birthday colleagues and friends collaborated to produce a special birthday volume of the (British) *Journal of Bone and Joint Surgery* (February 1956). Fairbank achieved all this, with a knighthood in 1946 for his administrative work in the Second World War, while conducting a busy private practice at 84 Harley Street, and at the same time completing his classic and enduring work entitled *Atlas of General Affections of the Skeleton*. He also handed down what might well be a unique distinction: not only did his son become a distinguished orthopaedic surgeon but his grandson, too, follows the same career, in the third generation.

Partial rapprochement

General surgeons and orthopaedic surgeons eventually came together at the Royal Society of Medicine in Wimpole Street in July 1925, when the sections of surgery and of orthopaedics of the Society held a joint meeting under the dual chairmanship of Sir Berkeley Moynihan, the well known general surgeon of Leeds (for the Society's Section of Surgery), and Professor E. W. Hey Groves, a remarkably astute orthopaedic surgeon from Bristol (for the Section of Orthopaedics). The main subject for discussion was the treatment of fractures, which had long been a bone of contention between the two groups. General surgeons had always held that the treatment of fractures was their preserve, and they resented the intrusion of orthopaedic surgeons into this lucrative field. Even at that date (1925), when most of the London teaching hospitals had appointed orthopaedic surgeons to the staff, it became clear that there was still no uniformity of opinion and, indeed, that some acrimony remained.

The first speaker was Professor G. E. Gask, of St Bartholomew's Hospital in London, who said that he was opposed to the growing tide of specialism which first began when surgery was divorced from medicine by an edict of Pope Alexander III, in 1163. He believed that this artificial separation of the two great branches of the healing art was the greatest blow that had befallen the profession, and still constituted a weakness. He deplored any further separation: future efforts should be directed instead towards fusion. He was especially worried about the effect that any further specialisation would have on the teaching of students. He reminded the audience that the authorities at his own hospital (St Bartholomew's), after long discussion, had decided not to establish a separate department of urology: certain younger members of the staff would be encouraged to take up and teach this specialty as part of their ordinary work as general surgeons. He would like to see the same applied to fracture surgery.

Sir Robert Jones (Liverpool and London) countered by stating that the treatment of fractures was not as good as it should be, and that the great teaching hospitals should give a lead to better things. Fractures were regarded as an incubus in most of the general surgical wards: they were of little interest to the majority of general surgeons, whose house surgeons were encouraged to discharge the patients at the earliest possible moment to make room for patients who needed some form of operative treatment. The treatment of fractures in the outpatient department, which was left almost entirely to the inexpert resident staff, without any supervision by the surgeons themselves, was even worse. Lamentable deformities, which should not have arisen, often followed fractures treated at teaching hospitals. Sir Robert favoured the segregation of patients with fractures in special wards, though not necessarily under the care of a single surgeon: staffing of the department by more than one surgeon would lead to a healthy rivalry between them, with resulting benefit to both patient and surgeon.

A lively debate ensued, which revealed that there was still a deep division of opinion. Several general surgeons spoke in support of Professor Gask's views, deploring the segregation of patients with fractures in special units, whereas, in general, orthopaedic surgeons favoured the proposition put forward by Sir Robert Jones.

A moderating opinion came from Dr Robert Osgood, a visiting orthopaedic surgeon from Boston, Massachusetts, who said that a scheme of segregation of fractures as advocated by Sir Robert Jones had been in operation at his hospital for some years, and it had proved successful. Previously some fractures – in particular the not uncommon compression fracture of the spine – had gone unrecognised, and others had caused unnecessary crippling. As a result, a number of industrial companies had formed their own fracture clinics, and this had stimulated surgeons to act themselves. A speaker from Edinburgh agreed that the treatment of fractures in Britain was unsatisfactory and that there was a heavy financial cost to employers of labour.

In closing the meeting, Professor Hey Groves commented that there was virtual unanimity among the speakers that there was room for improvement in the present treatment of fractures. War experience had made surgeons dissatisfied with present results.

Royal Society of Medicine, 1 Wimpole Street

This meeting at the Royal Society of Medicine was typical of many meetings covering all the specialties in medicine. The Society was a suitable forum for all kinds of medical discussion. Founded in 1805 as the Medical and Chirurgical Society of London, it received its Royal Charter in 1834. In 1907 fourteen specialty societies were merged with it, and the new body was renamed the Royal Society of Medicine. It outgrew its original premises in Hanover Square, and a new building was commissioned in Wimpole Street, at the corner with Henrietta Place. This was completed in 1910 and the Society moved in during the next two years. At its new site, the Royal Society of Medicine was easily accessible to doctors living in Harley Street or Wimpole Street, or in the neighbouring area. Two centuries on from its foundation, and with one of the largest medical libraries in Europe, it still serves a valuable purpose, and after further extension in 1982–86 and radical refurbishment in 2004–05 it now caters for large audiences in the 300-seat auditorium, and also provides residential and club facilities. The Society also has a long lease on Chandos House, the elegant eighteenth-century mansion in Chandos Street, close to Harley Street. This is used for major functions, and it provides additional accommodation for members of the Society.

Ophthalmology: Sir John Tweedy

From orthopaedic surgery to the very delicate specialty of ophthalmology. This was well represented in the heyday of Harley Street practice by Sir John Tweedy (1849–1934), who lived and practised at 100 Harley Street. Tweedy became distinguished not only as an ophthalmic surgeon on the staff of the Royal London Ophthalmic Hospital at Moorfields, but also, later in life, as an editor of *The Lancet*, the medical journal founded in 1823. In addition to his appointment at Moorfields he was also elected as assistant surgeon at University College Hospital, and from 1888 until 1904 he was Professor of Ophthalmology at University College, while still continuing his work at Moorfields. As editor of *The Lancet*, Tweedy served at a difficult time, when there was antipathy between that journal and certain members of hospital staffs. By virtue of his transparent honesty and a large measure of tact, he was able largely to convert enemies into friends.

Tweedy's growing popularity led to his election in 1892 to the Council of the Royal College of Surgeons of England; and after eleven years on the Council he was elected President of the College for a term of three years, from 1903. At the termination of this office he received the honour of knighthood (1906).

Like all those who prove good at administration and enjoy it, Tweedy was in great demand for his services from many professional bodies. Among the many positions that he accepted were the presidency of the Royal Medical Benevolent Fund and of the Medico-Legal Society. He had the advantage, in his many writings – especially for *The Lancet* – of being a first-class Latin scholar, with also a sound knowledge of Greek. In recognition of his wide knowledge of history and of the arts he was elected as Master of the Worshipful Company of Barbers, a livery company that was closely associated with the surgeons until their separation as the Company of Surgeons in 1745.

Famous physicians

The emphasis up to this point has been on surgery and surgeons, rather than on physicians. Between the two World Wars, two London physicians acquired huge reputations and were very much in the public eye. Both were raised to the peerage. They lived respectively in Wimpole Street and Harley Street. They were Lord Dawson of Penn and Lord Horder of Ashford.

Lord Dawson of Penn

Bertrand Dawson (1864–1945) was the son of an architect and was born in Purley, near Croydon, Surrey. He attended St Paul's School in London before proceeding to University College for further education, gaining a BSc degree in 1888. He studied medicine at the London Hospital, where he qualified in 1890 and became MD three years later. He was appointed as assistant physician to the London Hospital in 1896 and became full physician in 1906.

So far, a fairly usual start to a career. But in 1910 Dawson was appointed as physician extra-ordinary to the Royal Household. And in 1914 he was promoted to physician-in-ordinary to King George V. These appointments redirected his whole career. Accompanying the King to the war front in France as consulting physician to the army, he noticed the poor medical condition of the troops. This observation impelled him to make a study of trench fever, which was a cause of major disablement in the First World War. Later, as chairman of the Consultative Council on Medical and Allied Services, he submitted a report (1920) which foreshadowed the structure of the National Health Service, introduced by Aneurin Bevan in 1948. In 1920 he was appointed to the peerage as Baron Dawson of Penn, and thereafter he took an active part in the proceedings of the House of Lords. He became a viscount in 1936.

Dawson was acclaimed in 1928 when he attended King George V for a severe attack of pneumonia, complicated by a purulent infection which necessitated pleural drainage. He was credited with having saved the King's life. He carried on a lucrative private practice at 32 Wimpole Street, but quite early in his career he curtailed his practice in order to concentrate on hospital work and teaching. He again came into the limelight in 1936, when King George V lay dying at Sandringham, in Norfolk. Dawson was called in on 17 January, and a day or so later he issued a now famous statement: 'The King's life is moving peacefully towards its close'. George V died on 20 January.

Lord Dawson might not have received the universal respect that he did at that time if the true facts relating to the King's death had been known. For it turned out that death had been hastened by an injection of morphia and cocaine, administered to the comatose monarch by Dawson himself. The truth did not become public until fifty years later, when Lord Dawson's private diaries were opened. It was then revealed that Dawson, without consulting two other doctors involved in the case, decided that the King's death should be hastened, ostensibly to ease the pressure upon the family:

> At about 11 o'clock [p.m.] it was evident that the last stage might endure for many hours, unknown to the patient but little comporting with the dignity and serenity which he so richly merited and which demanded a brief final scene. Hours of waiting just for the mechanical end, when all that is really life has departed, only exhausts the onlookers and keeps them so strained that they cannot avail themselves of the solace of thought, communion or prayer. I therefore decided to determine the end, and injected (myself) morphia gr. ¾ and, shortly afterwards, cocaine gr. 1 into the distended jugular vein.

It is recorded that Sister Catherine Black, from the London Hospital, who had nursed the King during an illness in 1928, was present and had been asked to give the fatal injection, but she had refused to do so; and therefore Dawson gave it himself. (In an autobiography that she wrote late in life, Sister Black did not mention the incident.) The diaries revealed that the real reason for Dawson's having accelerated the King's death was to enable the news of the death to be published in the most respectable morning paper, *The Times*, rather than in the less appropriate evening papers. Also, having issued a statement that death was near, Dawson was concerned to show that his prognostication had been correct. In retrospect, his conduct seems to have been arrogant, to say the least, though understandable.

As was usual among doctors who had attained high rank, Lord Dawson of Penn received innumerable honours. He was chairman of many medico-political bodies, and President of the Royal College of Physicians for seven years, an unusually long term of office. He was also much concerned with the health and well-being of the ordinary person – of the nation as a whole – not only with his own patients. He was strongly in favour of birth control (as contraception was called at that time) and he opposed the many campaigns that were mounted against it. His views come over as modern even by today's standards:

> Sex love is one of the clamant, dominating forces of the world. Here we have an instinct, so fundamental, so imperious that its influence is a fact which has to be accepted: suppress it you cannot. You may guide it into healthy channels but an outlet it will have; and if that outlet is inadequate or unduly obstructed, irregular channels will be forced. All are agreed that union of body should be in association with union of mind and soul; all are agreed that the rearing of children is the pre-eminent purpose. But has not sexual union over and over again been the physical expression of our love without thought or intention of procreation?… Sex love has, apart from parenthood, a purport of its own. It is an essential part of health and happiness in

marriage. If sexual union is a gift from God it is worth learning how to use it.… It should be cultivated so as to bring physical satisfaction to both, not merely to one. The attainment of mutual and reciprocal joy in their relations constitutes a firm bond between two people and makes for durability of their marriage tie.…

Birth control is here to stay. It is an established fact, and for good or evil to be accepted. No denunciations will abolish it. The reasons which lead parents to limit their offspring are sometimes selfish, but more often honourable and cogent: the desire to marry and to rear children well equipped for life's struggle. Limited incomes, the cost of living, and burdensome taxation are forcible motives. Furthermore, amongst the educated classes there is the desire of women to take part in life and their husbands' careers, which is incompatible with oft-recurring pregnancies. Absence of birth control means late marriages, and these carry with them irregular unions and all the baneful consequences. 'But', say many, 'birth control may be necessary, but the only birth control which is justifiable is voluntary abstention.' Such abstention would be either ineffective or, if effective, impracticable and harmful to health and happiness. To limit the size of a family to, say, four children, would be to impose on a married couple an amount of abstention which for long periods would almost be equivalent to celibacy; and the abstention would have to be most strict during the earlier years of married life, when desires are strongest. I maintain [that] a demand is being made which, for the most of people, it is impossible to meet; and that endeavours to meet it would impose a strain hostile to health and happiness, and carry with them grave dangers to morals. The thing is preposterous. You might as well put water by the side of a man suffering from thirst and tell him not to drink it. No; birth control by abstention is either ineffective, or, if effective, is pernicious. [Birth control] is said to be unnatural and intrinsically immoral. Civilisation involves the chaining of natural forces and their conversion to man's will and uses. When anaesthetics were first used in childbirth there was an outcry that their use was unnatural and wicked because God meant women to suffer. It is no more unnatural to control childbirth by artificial means than it is to halt consciousness during labour or for an operation. The use of childbirth control is good; its abuse bad.

Lord Horder of Ashford

Thomas Jeeves Horder (1871–1955) was almost of the same generation as Lord Dawson of Penn. Like Dawson, at the prime of his career he was raised to the peerage. But the two men were of very different character.

Horder was not acclaimed for any particular innovation or description of disease, but through his exceptional clinical acumen and his strong personality he gained a huge reputation. Much in demand from the aristocracy, he became the rich man's doctor. Later he served the Royal Family as extra physician to King George VI and Queen Elizabeth II. He was the quintessential 'society doctor' – one of the last of the breed. He was also a man of sharp contrasts: whereas he was demanding in pursuit of high fees for his private consultations, he would often waive his fee altogether if he regarded a particular patient as a 'deserving case'.

Born in 1871 at Shaftesbury in Dorset, the son of Albert Horder, Thomas was said in *Who's Who?* to have been educated 'privately', but this seems to have been somewhat erroneous, for in fact he attended Swindon High School. He studied medicine in London at St Bartholomew's Hospital, where he qualified in 1893 and gained the degree of MD in 1897. He became interested in pathology and for seven years was in charge of the post-mortem room at Bart's, overseeing more than 1,000 post-mortem examinations a year. This post gave him a valuable insight into the features of bodily disease and a solid base for clinical study. As he stated himself, 'autopsies are the bedrock of diagnosis'. He became highly regarded as a physician, and in due course he was appointed as physician to St Bartholomew's Hospital.

With his background in morbid anatomy, Horder soon became famous for his keen promotion of clinical pathology, a subject that had not been developed as rapidly as it should have been. He became well known for his practice of carrying out clinico-pathological examinations in the wards. His friend Sir William Osler, the world-famous physician, dubbed him 'the man who took the laboratory to the bedside'. He carried with him a case with syringes and other items for collecting samples of blood, urine or excreta from the patient: this became famous as 'Horder's box'. He wrote a textbook entitled *Clinical Pathology in Practice*, followed by *Essentials of Medical Diagnosis*.

Apart from his clinical work and his busy private practice at 141 Harley Street, Horder was active in a number of sociological causes that were the subject of hot debate at the time. He boldly supported the practice of abortion when there were valid reasons for it. 'Who knows better than the family doctor the dysgenic effects of Mrs Smith's rapidly repeated confinements, both on herself and on her children?'

More controversial was his support for eugenics, the science that appertains to the production of fine offspring. The subject is seldom discussed today – perhaps because it has associations with Adolf Hitler – but it was a live issue in the years between the two World Wars. Horder became associated with the Eugenics Society of Great Britain in 1924 and was its President from 1935 to 1944. He regarded eugenics as a logical step in preventing the ravages of disease and improving the quality of life for future generations. In his *Fifty Years of Medicine* he wrote: 'In the view of the eugenist – a view which I share with utter conviction – the economic advantages, using the term in its widest sense, lie with efforts made toward racial betterment rather than with social service in a particular generation'.

Horder favoured voluntary sterilisation of carriers of hereditable disease. He was also an advocate of cremation in preference to burial, at a time when cremation was not common practice.

Horder was much in demand as chairman or president of medical and socio-logical organisations, some of which he founded. Among these were the British Empire Cancer Campaign and the Empire Rheumatism Council. He was sometime President of the Section of Medicine of the Royal Society of Medicine, and of the Harveian Society of London.

After the Second World War, in which Horder served as a medical adviser to government departments, there was active debate on the merits of establishing a health service to cover everyone in the land. Horder was opposed to such 'socialised medicine'. He founded the Fellowship of Medicine, which attracted 900 doctors who were antipathetic to a national scheme. Their efforts, of course, were in vain: there was strong support for Aneurin Bevan, the Minister of Health, when in 1948 his proposals for the National Health Service were put into effect.

Thomas Horder was knighted in 1918 and was created a baronet in 1923. Ten years later, in 1933, he was created Baron Horder of Ashford, and was thereafter known as Lord Horder. For many years he was also Deputy Lieutenant for the County of Hampshire.

Lord Horder was the last of a succession of Harley Street personalities who became famous because of their public appeal. Such men became household names and their statements and activities were always newsworthy. After the Second World War, the interest of the public in doctors generally, and particu-larly in 'society physicians', began to fade, as the number of specialists steadily increased and they were absorbed into the National Health Service rather than airing their views from Harley Street.

Chapter 6

A change of character

The character of early practice

In the early decades after doctors moved into Harley Street, unexpired leases on the houses, many with more than fifty years still to run, were purchased by individual doctors. The ground floor was given over to the medical practice, with consulting room, waiting room and one or two rooms for the secretaries. Often there was need for more than one secretary, for in the days before electronic communication the handling of records, letters and reports was painstaking and time consuming. With all this activity, Harley Street houses were by no means too large for their purpose.

The surgeon or physician lived in some degree of elegance. He would be decked out in frock coat and white spats, and when out of doors with silk top hat; and he would be attended by his butler or manservant. His wife, mistress of the house, looked after the servants below stairs. Although the servants' quarters were dingy and their work uncongenial as well as dirty, a kind mistress could ease their lot. Otherwise, the staff tended to change rather more often than would be wished. On his outside visits, the doctor would travel in his carriage and pair, or in a victoria or brougham, attended by the groom or grooms, who usually lived in quarters above the stable, in the mews at the rear of the property. A successful physician or surgeon might well have to maintain a staff of eight to ten people, depending upon his commitments.

The beginning of multiple tenancies

This system continued with little change until the early years of the twentieth century: it was the declining lifestyle of the Victorian era, with its severe consciousness of class. But gradually a few consultants, while continuing to practise in Harley Street itself or in the immediate vicinity, chose to live elsewhere, either in one of the nearby villages, such as St John's Wood, Primrose Hill or Hampstead, or further afield, in the rapidly growing suburbs. This trend became more pronounced during and after the First World War, as doctors became aware of the advantages of living away from the practice, in an area where the family felt less 'closed in' than in Harley Street, and as travelling became easier with the demise of the horse-drawn vehicle and the adoption of motor transport. Hampstead was perhaps the most popular location. An example of one of those who moved out there was William Trethowan, a successful orthopaedic surgeon on the staff of Guy's Hospital, with a lucrative practice at 134 Harley Street. A talented musician, he had a large organ installed in his house in Hampstead, where he would often play well into the night. The house also had a large garden – another major attraction of properties outside central London.

Subject to the agreement of the ground landlord, a consultant who lived away from Harley Street but continued to practise there was in a position to sublet rooms to other doctors for consulting: and thus began the system of multiple tenancies, with up to three or four doctors (later, often even more) working in a single house. This new trend began slowly, with the first multiple tenancies established at about the end of the nineteenth century. But it advanced rapidly in the first decades of the twentieth century, especially after the First World War. Thereafter fewer and fewer consultants actually lived and worked under the same roof. There were, of course, a few die-hards who continued to practise from their Harley Street homes and to live there as well: some resisted change right up to the time of the Second World War.

This fundamental change in the original system of Harley Street practice really signalled the end of the glamour that had attached to Harley Street and its doctors. With the number of practitioners growing rapidly, and ever fewer of them actually residing in Harley Street, consultants tended to lose their individuality: they became part of the crowd. It was the end of the 'Harley Street era'.

Harley Street today

At the present time, Harley Street houses are occupied almost entirely in the daytime by medical men or women in every type of specialty, with many dentists as well; and by ancillary staff such as psychologists, physiotherapists and practitioners of so-called complementary medicine. In recent years there has also been a sprinkling of lawyers practising among the doctors, almost entirely at the southern end of Harley Street. A small proportion of these people may live in flats in the upper storeys or basements; but most live outside, often many miles away from Harley Street, and travel in daily to their work. An army of cleaners arrives in the early morning or in the late evening; where they come from and where they go when their work is done is not well recorded. At night Harley Street and the adjacent streets often seem sadly deserted.

With approximately 150 houses in the street, and with an average of perhaps four practitioners in each, the total number of professionals working there may be estimated as well over 600. Similar estimates would apply to Wimpole Street, with its northern extensions Upper Wimpole Street and Devonshire Place, and there are scores more professional people working in the adjacent streets, especially Queen Anne Street and Weymouth Street. So the medical and para-medical population may be measured in thousands.

Properties in Harley Street and in adjacent streets were badly damaged by German bombs during the Second World War. Some terraces were demolished almost entirely, or were so badly damaged that they had to be pulled down. Even apart from war damage, many of the original houses have been greatly altered or totally rebuilt in a different style of architecture; there are now few houses that remain in their original state. Most of those in Harley Street that are reasonably well preserved are in the northern terraces, which were the last to be built. It is in these terraces, near the Marylebone Road, that one may still gain an impression of how Harley Street looked in its prime. Looking northwards from there, one still has a glimpse, between the opposing terraces, of green foliage in Regent's Park. Since 1835, when the Park was first opened to the public, it has been a delightful amenity for those living or working in the area.

Fading prestige

Apart from the gradual change in the character of Harley Street and Wimpole Street that took place when residential occupancy began to give place to multiple tenancies, there has also been a change in the prestige rating of different parts of the Harley Street area. In the early years, houses in or near Cavendish Square were the most highly prized, and leases there sold at a premium over properties further away. Indeed, so prestigious was Cavendish Square as an address that, even as late as the Second World War, residents or lessees of houses in Harley Street and thereabouts felt almost universally impelled to add 'Cavendish Square' to the actual address on their headed notepaper. Thus, a resident at, say, 25 Harley Street would list the address as 25 Harley Street, Cavendish Square, London W. This would apply not only to headed notepaper and to the telephone directory, but also to an entry in the Medical Directory.

The preference for Cavendish Square or the nearest that one could get to it has now gone into reverse. There is no longer any realistic opportunity for a doctor to practise in Cavendish Square itself: most of the houses there, except for a few on the north side, have long been replaced by modern premises dedicated to commercial rather than professional use. The favoured centre of professional practice has now shifted northwards, towards the Marylebone Road, with consulting suites at Number 149, the Harley Street wing of the London Clinic, being particularly favoured. One reason for this may be that the consulting suites there have the big advantage that ancillary services such as radiology, pathology and physiotherapy are immediately to hand in the same building. Indeed, the London Clinic, established in 1932, tends to dominate the north end both of Devonshire Place (where the main entrance is situated) and of Harley Street. There are other notable medical and nursing institutions in Harley Street – notably the Harley Street Clinic (with its entrance on Weymouth Street), an important centre for cardio-thoracic surgery.

It is not always appreciated that, even up till the time of the Second World War, the centre of medical specialisation in England remained firmly in London. It is true that there were specialist physicians and surgeons in provincial cities, but there were not many. Some were eminent enough to achieve national and international fame – for instance Sir Berkeley Moynihan (1865–1936) of Leeds, a widely acclaimed abdominal surgeon; and Sir Robert Jones (1858–1933), pioneer orthopaedic surgeon, of Liverpool (though later of London – see Chapter 6). In general, though, specialist branches of medicine and surgery, such as neurology, neurosurgery, thoracic surgery and orthopaedic surgery, were sparsely represented outside London. Thus, patients seeking a specialist opinion in such fields generally had to make their way to London or, if they could afford it, to have a London specialist visit them.

All this changed after the Second World War, with the introduction of the National Health Service in 1948. Increasingly from then on, medical institutions in major cities and even in smaller towns sought to establish specialist departments in nearly every branch of medicine and surgery; and it was not long before the standard of care in these special branches was equal to the best available in London.

Quite apart from the physical changes that have been described, there has been a change in the public perception of Harley Street and of the doctors who practise there. In the heyday of Harley Street, at about the turn of the nineteenth century with the twentieth, there was an indefinable 'glamour' surrounding medical specialists, whether they were physicians, surgeons or experts in other fields of medicine. Charismatic doctors often became household names, and their treatment of aristocratic patients, and especially of royalty, was often headline news in the daily press.

In those class-conscious times it was relatively common for well favoured specialists to achieve distinction through the honour of a knighthood, or even a baronetcy, and a privileged few (beginning with Lord Lister, the first medical baron) were elevated to the peerage.

The change that occurred in this public appraisal of doctors, and of the awards that were made to them by the authorities, was a relatively sudden one. It happened almost immediately after the establishment of the National Health Service in 1948. At a stroke, the number of consultants who entered hospital practice was increased dramatically. Moreover, they now received reasonable payment for their services, whereas previously most consultants, with no more than 'honorary' hospital appointments, had had to rely upon fees from their private practice to make ends meet. A few physicians and surgeons became wealthy but, contrary to what is generally imagined, in the early days of Harley Street specialists often found it difficult to get established in practice unless they had independent means. They sought hospital appointments not because such posts were lucrative (the reverse was the case, for consultants often gave their services free), but because attachment to a hospital might bring an enviable reputation that would be reflected in a demand for private consultations. Before the National Health Service came into being, even junior doctors, who were not able to practise privately, received derisory salaries for their hospital work. In the 1930s and 1940s, £100 or £150 per year was the usual remuneration for resident junior staff. At a prestigious institution such as a London teaching hospital they received nothing more than free board and lodging during their first appointments. They were willing to accept such stringency and to work all hours because of the training that they received.

With the large increase in the number of specialists after the Second World War and the start of the National Health Service, there was noticeable dilution of perquisites that went with successful practice; a much smaller proportion of specialists were selected for awards such as knighthoods, and medical baronets were no longer created. At the same time, the public's perception of a doctor's stature gradually diminished. The glamour of elite medicine and surgery had gone. The heyday of Harley Street had lasted little more than half a century – from the 1890s until 1948, when it was killed by the introduction of the National Health Service.

The popular press has replaced coverage of elite medicine and its practitioners with almost daily revelations of alleged 'advances' that 'could' achieve this or that breakthrough, in five or ten years' time. (Or they might not.) They have to make headlines. Harley Street has become irrelevant amid real developments that have taken place in universities and progressive hospitals throughout the country. A Harley Street address no longer means very much – if anything at all. There are bad doctors there, as well as good doctors. Yet a certain glamour does still linger on. It will take time to die. Today, what really matters is expertise, no matter where its possessor may practise. It may be in Harley Street; or it may be in Nottingham, Wigan or Bristol; or elsewhere in London. A difficulty for the ordinary patient, seeking the best treatment, is to find out where to go.

Chapter 7

Historical notes on the development of Regent's Park

The place for a park

In the early years of Harley Street, residents were fortunate in having easy access to the country. Until the early years of the nineteenth century there was open country immediately to the north, where local people could walk in fields still grazed by cattle and sheep (see Figure 3, p. 15). There were pleasant rural tea gardens and country taverns within a few minutes' walk – notably the Jew's Harp tea garden and the tavern known as the Queen's Head and Artichoke, which still exists, though on a new site, in Albany Street. From the upper end of Harley Street and Devonshire Place there was an uninterrupted view across the country towards Hampstead and Highgate.

This pleasant rural environment suffered from gradual encroachment as the built-up area around Harley Street crept gradually northwards in the nineteenth century. But, in recompense, residents were soon to enjoy the elegant amenities of Regent's Park, mostly completed by 1828 but not opened to the public until a few years later. It was at first closed to the public in the interests of residents: only the roads were open to all. This restriction was eased in 1835, when public access was allowed to a large area of the open ground. In 1841 access was further eased, to the extent that only small areas were reserved for the sole benefit of residents, mainly in the immediate vicinity of the villas and terraces. As recently as the years after the Second World War, commercial vehicles were prohibited from travelling through the park, and traffic was controlled by local speed restrictions.

Access to the park became an even greater asset for later generations of the public, when open country receded many miles away. Regent's Park then became a playground for a multitude of people, with facilities provided for many sports, including football, hockey, tennis and boating, and with safe play areas for young children.

It was largely a matter of good fortune that Regent's Park as we know it today came into being. When plans to develop the Crown land that had been Marylebone Park were first mooted at the turn of the eighteenth century, it was 'touch and go' as to whether the area would be swallowed up in a criss-cross grid of featureless streets and houses like those that had recently been constructed on neighbouring estates – the Portland estate, the Portman estate, the Bloomsbury estate. Projects for the development of just such a maze of streets had been submitted when suggestions had first been solicited. If such plans had been adopted, there would be no Regent's Park today. It was mainly through the clear-sighted intellect of a newly appointed civil servant that such a disaster was avoided and that the open space that is Regent's Park was preserved. That man was John Fordyce. He deserves wide recognition for his service to the nation.

John Fordyce

John Fordyce was born in 1735 in North Berwickshire, into a prominent Scottish land-owning family. His father had been involved in dealing, on behalf of a building company, with land forfeited after the Jacobite rebellion of 1745. John Fordyce succeeded to his father's estate when still a young man. In 1766 he became Receiver General of Land Revenues for Scotland. He was married to Catherine, daughter of Sir William Maxwell of Monteith, whose sister was the wife of the Duke of Gordon. Fordyce was thus a man of substance, experienced in land management, when in 1793 he was appointed as Surveyor General for Crown Lands in London. He was the right man for the job: enthusiastic, hard working and – most importantly – with a clear and wise insight into what was needed for the full development of the former Marylebone Park. He immediately saw the need for a fresh and detailed survey of the estate, the rental from which had been shrinking steadily since the restoration of the monarchy in 1660.

Fordyce appreciated that the park was rather far from central parts of London such as Westminster, the Houses of Parliament and the Law Courts, for houses there to be greatly in demand. He foresaw that property values would be much enhanced if travel to and from the centre of London could be speeded up. 'The best, and ... the most advantageous way of doing that would be by opening a great street from Charing Cross towards a central part of Marylebone Park'. Fordyce envisaged a newly developed park served by this projected new road (Regent Street), which he emphasised should be not less than seventy feet wide. He accepted that the construction of the road would necessitate the demolition of substantial areas of existing housing, but he regarded this as a price to be paid. He probably already had in mind the architect who could best undertake the design of this vast project – John Nash.

John Nash

The second key figure in the development of Regent's Park was indeed the dynamic architect John Nash. Born in 1752, Nash was already past middle age and with wide experience when he was instructed to prepare an overall plan for the development of a new park and for the construction of a wide new road to link that park with Westminster.

Nash had studied architecture under the supervision of Sir Robert Taylor. By the time he came to be involved in the development of Regent's Park he had been in practice for many years and had designed many country houses, mainly for clients in Wales and on the Isle of Wight, where he had his own house. He had inherited money from an uncle and had retired to Wales, but financial difficulties culminating in bankruptcy forced him to rebuild his career.

Nash had the ability to envisage the wider picture presented by his briefs, leaving less important details aside. This was a valuable trait when it came to laying out the wide expanse of land that had been Marylebone Park, and to planning an entirely new road across London. He was criticised for the use of painted stucco on nearly all his buildings in the park, as a cheaper alternative to the use of Portland stone. But not everyone regarded this as a fault. There were, and still are, many who find that the stuccoed buildings bring a sense of air and light to the estate, especially since many of the buildings are set in open spaces generously planted with trees and shrubs, often within sight of open water. Nash also had the advantage of having collaborated for some years with Humphry Repton, one of the most acclaimed landscape gardeners of the time. Together they had designed country estates where the house blended well with the surrounding acres to form a 'picturesque' whole. Nash profited from this experience when he came to lay out individual villas in such a way that they seemed to lie in a wooded country setting, whereas in fact they were not far away from other buildings.

Repton may also have been responsible for introducing Nash to the Prince of Wales, as he was before becoming Prince Regent in 1811 and King George IV in 1820. As early as 1798 Nash had designed a conservatory for the Prince, who himself had a lifelong enthusiasm for architecture. He had commissioned Nash to design the Royal Pavilion in Brighton, and he was later to instruct him to convert Buckingham House in London to form Buckingham Palace.

After the death of John Fordyce in 1809 the affairs of the Crown lands were entrusted to three newly appointed Commissioners of Woods and Forests (Crown Commissioners), who were to be responsible for all decisions, subject to the approval of the Treasury. Two architects appointed by the Commissioners were John Nash and James Morgan. Nash was clearly the prime mover; Morgan was barely more than a 'sleeping partner'.

It was in 1810, a year after the death of John Fordyce, that the Commissioners formally instructed their surveyors and their architects, Nash and Morgan, to draw up plans for the redevelopment of the old Marylebone Park, and for the linking road that was to become Regent Street. It was stipulated that the park should be a residential area for the more substantial members of the community. There was also to be a barracks and a new church to serve the parishioners of Marylebone. The Prince Regent was keenly interested in the whole project, later lending his title to 'Regent's Park'. He steadfastly supported Nash throughout, even when difficult problems arose.

It had been many years since Marylebone Park had ceased to be the hunting ground that it had become after Henry VIII took it over in 1539, at the dissolution of the monasteries. It had been desecrated as a park by Cromwell during the Commonwealth. After the restoration of the monarchy in 1660 the land was let out for farming. At the turn of the eighteenth century it was simply part of the general countryside, with nothing to mark it out as a park: even the boundaries had disappeared. There were three tenanted farms, with associated farm buildings. In the eastern sector there were the tea gardens already mentioned – the Jew's Harp – and the Queen's Head and Artichoke. This was the Crown land that was to become the Regent's Park.

When Nash submitted his plans (with little or no input from Morgan), he included a detailed report in which he set out the principles that had dictated his design. His prose reflects the verbosity of speech and quaint punctuation of the time. It is worth quoting from his report. He recommended:

> that Mary-le-Bone Park shall be made to contribute to the health-fulness, beauty, and advantage, of that quarter of the Metropolis: that the houses and buildings to be erected shall be of that useful description, and permanent construction, and shall possess such local advantages, as shall be likely to assure a great augmentation of revenue to the Crown at the expiration of the leases; that the attraction of open space, free air and the scenery of Nature, with the means and invitation of exercise on horseback, on foot and in carriages, shall be preserved or created in Mary-le-Bone Park, as allurements or motives for the wealthy part of the Public to establish themselves there; and that the advantages which the circumstances of the situation itself present shall be improved and advanced; and that markets, and conveniences essential to the comforts of Life shall be placed in situa-tions, and under such circumstances, as may induce tradesmen to settle there.

Detailing his plans, Nash stated that the park was to be a residential area approached only from Baker Street, Devonshire Place and Portland Place. There was to be no entrance from the poorer estates, on the west and east sides. At the entrance from Portland Place there was to be a large circus, with the parish church in the middle. There was to be a double circus in the centre of the park. A drive fifty feet wide was to be constructed at the periphery, extending to two-thirds of the circumference, with terraces of houses on its outer side, facing inwards towards the centre. In the north there was to be a barracks for the

Lifeguards and Artillery. The interior was to remain as open parkland, with fifty-six individual villas blended in with the landscape, and secluded so far as possible from the view of the others. A larger villa was to be designed with a view to its occupation by the Prince Regent.

In the east, away from the main residential precincts, there was to be a service area in which small houses would be built for tradesmen. There would be three separate markets, for meat, hay and vegetables. The service area and the barracks were to be separated from the residential area by a canal, which would provide cheap water-borne transport for merchandise and would enhance the scenic vista.

The park was to be linked to the Westminster area by the new wide road (Regent Street) that had been proposed by John Fordyce. Essentially this would be a southward extension of Portland Place, which would form the northernmost quarter mile of the route. The road would continue southwards to its crossing with Oxford Street, where there would be a circus (Oxford Circus). There would be another circus (Piccadilly Circus) at the crossing with Piccadilly. Thence the road would open up a route (Lower Regent Street) towards Carlton House, the residence of the Prince Regent. The road south of Oxford Street was to be so located as to separate the prestigious area around Hanover Square, to the west, from the poorer area of Soho, in the east.

Nash had substantially overestimated the revenue that would accrue to the Crown from ground rents, and he had underestimated the costs that would be incurred. This became painfully evident within the first few years of the venture; but Nash was not deterred, and the Prince Regent continued his support.

Nash's plans were well received by the Commissioners, who liked the general concept of blending town-style houses into a country-style setting. But his design was not accepted in its entirety: substantial modifications were demanded. First, it was stipulated that the peripheral drive should encircle the park completely, rather than being restricted to two-thirds of the perimeter. (This was a sensible amendment, insisted upon by Lord Glenbervie, the chief Commissioner.) Secondly, it was thought that there were too many villas in Nash's design. They were to be reduced from fifty-six to twenty-six. (In the event, only eight villas were built.) Furthermore, it was demanded that the barracks should be on the eastern section of the park, near the area set aside for the tradesmen and markets. And lastly, it was stipulated that the canal should be sited at the edge of the park, on the east side, away from the open area in which Nash had placed it for its scenic value. (It was not thought desirable that bargees should intrude into the residential area.) Nash was disappointed by this amendment, which he thought deprived the park of the attractiveness of water; but he had to accept it.

Subject to revision of the plans along these lines, the go-ahead for the development was given in October 1811, which is thus marked as the year in which Regent's Park was initiated. The first step was to be the plantation of trees and shrubs and the construction of the perimeter drive. Work on these projects started almost immediately. Notice to leave was given to the tenants of farms and buildings. The principal farmer, Thomas Willan, objected to being turned out, but he nevertheless packed up and moved to West Twyford, in Middlesex, where he continued to prosper. The landlords of the Jew's Harp tea rooms and the Queen's Head and Artichoke public house took new leases near the eastern edge of the park, whereupon their original buildings were demolished.

Clearance of the land allowed the route of the perimeter drive to be marked out. Within a year construction of the drive was almost complete, and most of the trees and shrubs had been planted. Some leases had been taken up for building sites, mainly in the eastern section of the park, near the site of the markets. But as late as five years into the project the Commissioners had to report that the expenditure, then standing at £53,650, had already been more than four times the amount that Nash had estimated. Take-up of leases in the residential area had been disappointing, and very little building had begun. Unforeseen problems had been caused by the wars with France, which had led to marked depression in the building industry. Thus, the whole project was proving to be much more difficult than had been expected.

Construction of the canal, in particular, caused huge problems for Nash, who had a personal financial interest in the project. There was difficulty, first, in deciding the course of the canal from its origin at the Grand Junction Canal in Paddington, to its entry into the Thames at Limehouse. Landowners were reluctant to sell except with stringent stipulations. Thus, in the Maida Vale area it was demanded that only high-quality houses should be built on the banks. There was also difficulty in finding a source of water from which to maintain the level in the canal. Nash himself was unfazed by the difficulties, despite his having to take up all the leases for wharfs in the Regent's Park basin. At long last the Regent's Canal was opened with due ceremony in August 1820, eight years after its inception in a Parliamentary Bill passed in 1812. Nash's contribution to its achievement was applauded in *The Times*, as well as by the general public.

Another major problem that inhibited progress was related to the proposed circus at the north end of Portland Place, at its crossing with the New Road (Marylebone Road). A lease for the construction of houses in the circus had been taken by Charles Mayor, an entrepreneur and a business associate of Nash. Mayor claimed to be an architect himself and had erected houses in other parts of London. He started to build up the south-east quadrant of what was to be the circus, but long before the houses were finished money ran out and he became bankrupt. Building ceased and the houses stood unroofed and derelict; after a fire one of the houses collapsed and it remained for months as a ruin. Eventually the plans had to be revised: the concept of a full circus was abandoned in favour of a crescent in the south (now Park Crescent) and a square (Park Square) on the north side of the New Road (Marylebone Road). In due course, new lessees were found; Mayor's dilapidated relics were removed and handsome houses were constructed. But this had been a major setback.

Another serious difficulty arose over the proposed new church, which in Nash's original plan was to have been in the centre of the circus. Where was it to be sited now that the circus had been abandoned? Members of the vestry could not agree among themselves whether it should be in the remaining (south) crescent or whether it should be inside the park. The situation was further complicated when the Duke of Portland demanded that the church be built on his land. He declared that he would not allow the railings that closed the north end of Portland Place to be removed unless this was agreed, and unless the railings were removed there could be no access for vehicles between the park and Portland Place – an essential feature of Nash's plan.

As it happened, the Church authorities had already commissioned the building of a new 'chapel of ease' on the Marylebone Road, close to the old church of St Mary on Marylebone High Street, which had replaced an earlier church in 1741. To solve the dilemma they now changed course and gave instructions that a new parish church be erected on the site, instead of the chapel of ease. Thomas Hardwick was the architect: he designed the handsome building that is now the Marylebone parish church, facing the Marylebone Road (see Figure 10, p. 26). The church was consecrated in 1817.

John Nash took advantage of these changes to redesign the south entrance to Regent's Park, creating what is now one of his masterpieces, York Gate. This replaced the south entrance that he had originally planned, from Devonshire Place.

The many setbacks that were encountered were in part a reflection of the unlucky timing of the start of the development. But soon after a down-beat progress report had been submitted by the Commissioners in 1819, the situation was dramatically reversed. A period of prosperity began and there was a huge boom in house building. Within a few months nearly all the leases had been taken up, and construction was proceeding apace. One of the first projects to be completed was Park Crescent, which had been started early but had faltered badly in mid-term, as already described. Clearance for the route of Regent Street was also well advanced and much of the building work was complete by 1820. At that time, the long edifice of Cornwall Terrace was begun. Next came York Terrace near the Marylebone Road, Clarence Terrace and Sussex Place, with Park Square completed in 1823 and Hanover Terrace in 1826. The last terraces to be built were Chester Terrace and Cumberland Terrace, on the east side of the park, and Gloucester Gate, close to the north-east entrance.

This was a massive programme of building, especially when one considers that several of the country-style villas were going up at the same time; and soon to come was the erection of buildings in the new Zoological Gardens. Only in about 1828 was a respite called, when the Commissioners cancelled the construction of the two terraces planned for the north section of the park, namely Munster Terrace and Carrick Terrace.

Most of the buildings in the park were erected in the decade between 1818 and 1827. Nash oversaw the general design of all the terraces and was responsible himself or gave his approval for all the facades. In a few instances he was personally responsible for all the working drawings, notably for Sussex Place and Hanover Terrace. Nearly all the houses were built by speculative builders, who took a lease on a peppercorn rent while the house was being erected, but sold the house as soon as it was built, the tenant then taking a lease of ninety-nine years from the start of building. The cost of the lease was based on the length of the frontage, and it varied according to the amenities of the property. Thus, for York Terrace the cost was eighteen shillings per foot of frontage, whereas for Albany Street it was only ten shillings per foot.

Of the dozen or so builders who took part in the construction, the most prominent was James Burton. Wealthy already as a speculative builder, he took many of the leases and was responsible for the erection of more of the houses than any other builder. Nash also had a large personal financial interest in the park. Burton built for himself an attractive villa close to banks of the lake. The house was designed by his son Decimus, then only eighteen years old and probably dependent upon some help from his very experienced father in drawing up the plans. Trained under Nash's supervision, Decimus Burton was to design many other buildings in the park, as well as in other parts of London.

In a progress report of 1826, when much of the building in the park had been completed, the Commissioners stated that leases for eight of the proposed twenty-six villas had been taken up. In a surprise move, they then declared that no more villas would be built. Furthermore, they abandoned plans for a 'double circus' in the middle of the park, proposed by Nash: it had become a plain circular drive known as the Inner Circle. In their project-cutting shift of policy, the Commissioners had also called a halt to the construction of further terraces: they cancelled plans to build Munster Terrace and Carrick Terrace in the north part of the park, on the grounds that views towards Hampstead and Highgate in the north would be interrupted. Perhaps the gigantic scale of the project, with all the setbacks and complications that they had encountered, caused them to 'call it a day'.

The outcome of all these changes was that the appearance of the park when development was complete fell far short of what Nash had envisaged at the start (see Figure 13). Most of the alterations may well have been for the better; others were perhaps for the worse. Certainly there would have been much less open space if twenty-six villas had been built, as the Commissioners had first allowed, let alone the fifty-six planned by Nash. Either way, Regent's Park became one of the most beautiful parts of London, much admired by visitors from abroad as well as at home.

The villas

The eight villas that were finally built, out of the fifty-six that were originally intended by Nash, gave the park an air of rural peace and elegance. Mostly, they had the stature of small country houses set off by well planned plantations of trees and shrubs. Most were designed in the Greek classical style.

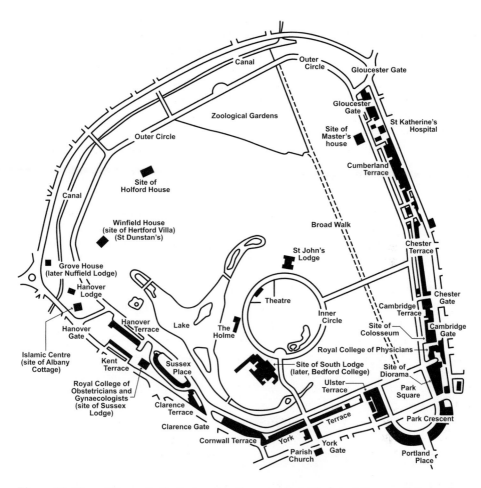

Figure 13 Plan of Regent's Park, showing the surviving Nash buildings and some of the historic sites. The Colosseum and the Diorama were both in the south-east corner of the park.

One of the first villas to be built, in 1818–19, was for occupation by James Burton, who, as already noted, was heavily involved in erecting other buildings in the park. It was known as The Holme (in Saxon, a river island) (Figure 14). Designed by Decimus Burton, his son, it stands close to the west rim of the Inner Circle. It is of medium size, with plan dimensions of 66 feet by 44 feet. There are two storeys above ground and a concealed basement. On the lakeside frontage there is a drawing room with a large window facing out over the water, flanked on one side by the library and on the other by a billiards room. The dining room and study are on the garden side. As was usual at the time, the kitchen and related offices were in the basement, concealed by shrubs and kept dry by area walls. The Burtons lived there until 1834. From 1913 to 1935 the villa was occupied by Sir George Dance, theatrical producer and song writer. After the Second World War the lease was taken by Bedford College (now Royal Holloway and Bedford New College), originally founded in Bedford Square, which was acquiring a substantial presence in Regent's Park. The Holme has now been restored for private occupation.

There were two other attractive villas on the perimeter of the Inner Circle. One of these, St John's Lodge, still stands, though not in its original form. It was designed for Charles Augustus Tulk, MP, by John Raffield, a Northumberland architect, who exhibited the design at the Royal Academy in 1818. From a slightly elevated position, the house commands extensive views across the park towards the zoo. As originally constructed, it had a dignified and elegant frontage, with large portico and symmetrical wings. A large arched window above the portico marked the second storey. This villa was extensively modified and enlarged in 1847 by the well known architect Charles Barry, and further enlarged for the third Marquess of Wellesley (eldest brother of the Duke of Wellington), Sir Izaac Lyon Goldsmid, philanthropist and one-time President of the Royal Society, and the Marquess of Bute. From 1921 to 1927 it was the headquarters of St Dunstan's Institute for the Blind. It was later taken over by Bedford College (as it then was) and called St John's Hall; but in the 1990s it reverted to private occupation, with the name St John's Lodge restored. A particularly attractive feature of this

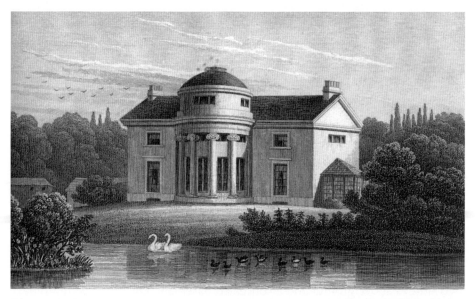

Figure 14 The Holme, designed by Decimus Burton for his father, James Burton, one of the most successful builders of Regent's Park. The house, on the lakeside, was one of the first villas to be built, and it was occupied by the Burton family for many years. From *London and Its Environs in the Nineteenth Century Illustrated by a Series of Views from Original Drawings by Thomas H. Shepherd* (London: James & Co., 1827).

property is the beautiful secluded garden, part of which is now open to the public, with access from the Inner Circle.

The third villa on the perimeter of the Inner Circle was known as South Villa (Figure 15). The architect is unknown. It was a fine building, with a pedimented Ionic portico supported on an arcaded loggia, and with bow windows on ground-floor and first-floor levels overlooking the park and the lake. For thirty years it was occupied by a wealthy wine merchant, George Bishop, who was prominent as an amateur astronomer, eventually becoming President of the Royal Astronomical Society. By permission of the Commissioners, he built an observatory in the Inner Circle, near the site of the present open-air theatre. After his death the observatory was moved to Twickenham, then – if no longer – a 'clean air' village. In 1908, the lease of South Villa was acquired by Bedford College, which had outgrown its accommodation in Bedford Square. The villa was later pulled down and replaced by the extensive academic buildings (then known as Bedford College) which now form a dominant feature of this part of the park, leaving a small octagonal porter's lodge as the only reminder of the original villa.

Other villas were built in the west and north-west part of the park. Albany Cottage (Figure 16), or North Villa, lay close behind Hanover Terrace. Described

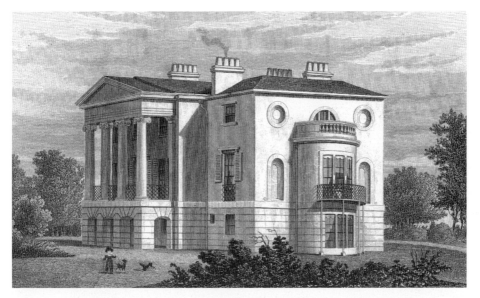

Figure 15 South Villa. The house had fine views over the park and the lake. It was demolished in the early years of the twentieth century to make way for Bedford College (now Royal Holloway and New Bedford College), which had outgrown its original premises in Bedford Square. From *London and Its Environs in the Nineteenth Century Illustrated by a Series of Views from Original Drawings by Thomas H. Shepherd* (London: James & Co., 1827).

as a *cottage ornée*, it was built in about 1827 for Thomas Raikes, City merchant, diarist and dandy. It was a two-storey building with the raised ground floor reached by a curved flight of steps. There was a pretty veranda, edged by large urns and a balustrade. This villa's tenants, over time, included William Myerstein, whose son Sir Edward Myerstein was a philanthropist and enormous benefactor to the Middlesex Hospital in London. The house was rebuilt between the two World Wars for Lady Ribblesdale, and it later became the headquarters of the Islamic Cultural Centre.

Hanover Lodge was a more elegant and larger house, said to have been designed by Nash himself. It had large reception rooms, nine bedrooms and a bathroom – an unusual luxury at the time. Like many of the villas, it had a handsome pedimented portico, embellished with four Doric columns, and a hall with marble columns and a tessellated floor. It was the home for a time of Admiral Lord Beatty, of Battle of Jutland fame in the First World War. Much altered, it was later leased by the French government as an ambassadorial residence. It has now been fully restored for renewed use as a private residence.

Hertford Villa, owned first by the Marquess of Hertford, was designed by Decimus Burton. It was the largest of the eight villas built in the park. A distinctive feature was the large portico, with six free-standing Corinthian pillars. The wings

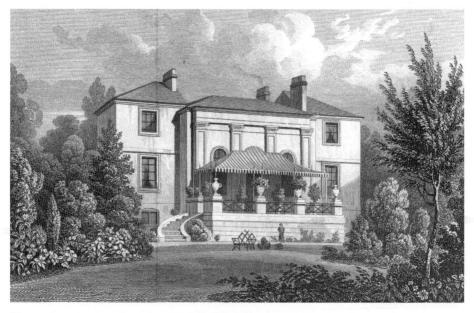

Figure 16 Albany Cottage, a neat small villa close to Hanover Gate on the west side of the park. It was replaced between the two world wars by a house built for Lady Ribblesdale, which later became the Islamic Cultural Centre. From *London and Its Environs in the Nineteenth Century Illustrated by a Series of Views from Original Drawings by Thomas H. Shepherd* (London: James & Co., 1827).

flanking the entrance each had three floor-to-ceiling windows. The second storey was placed further back, so that the front of each wing was only one storey high. The large dining room was noted for its elegance. The Marquess renamed the house St Dunstan's Villa, after St Dunstan's Church in Fleet Street, the unique clock from which he had salvaged and installed in his garden when the church was renovated. A later tenant, Lord Rothermere, restored the clock to its rightful place in St Dunstan's Church. Otto Hahn, an American banker who held the lease during the First World War, allowed the house to be used as a training centre for blinded soldiers and sailors, thus giving the name St Dunstan's to the charity. The villa was demolished in 1936 to make way for Winfield House, built for Barbara Hutton, grand-daughter of the founder of Woolworths. Winfield House later became the official residence of the Ambassador of the United States of America.

Grove House (Figure 17), another villa designed by Decimus Burton, was built in 1822–23 on the 'wrong' side of the Regent's canal, close to Prince Albert Road. It was a lavish house set in nearly three acres of ground. Through the portico there was a round hall leading to a rotunda with marble columns. The

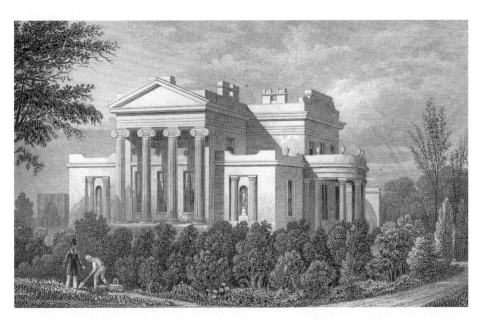

Figure 17 Grove House, a fine villa designed by Decimus Burton in 1822 for George Bellas Greenough, a scientist who was successively President of the Geological Society and the Geographical Society. It was later occupied by the artist Sigismund Goetze, who, among many benefactions, donated the gilded wrought iron gates at the entrance to Queen Mary's Gardens in the Inner Circle. From *London and Its Environs in the Nineteenth Century Illustrated by a Series of Views from Original Drawings by Thomas H. Shepherd* (London: James & Co., 1827).

ground-floor rooms comprised a large drawing room looking over the canal to the park, a large dining room, a billiards room and two libraries. Grove House was built for George Bellas Greenough, geologist and geographer, and one-time President both of the Geological Society and the Geographical Society. A later notable resident was Sigismund Goetze, a wealthy patron of the arts and a talented artist himself, who specialised in murals. He was a generous benefactor to the area in which he lived: the handsome gilded wrought iron gates at the entrance to Queen Mary's Gardens in the Inner Circle were a gift from Goetze and his wife, as also were two fountains in the gardens.

Holford House was another lavish villa, designed by Decimus Burton for James Holford, who, like an early tenant of South Villa, was a wealthy wine merchant. It was built after the other villas, in about 1832. Named after the occupant, Holford House was situated between Hertford House (St Dunstan's Villa) and the zoo, and was set in generous gardens. In its grandeur, the villa was the equal of Hertford House. The magnificent pedimented portico was flanked by semicircular bays at each side. For many years James Holford lived there alone, looked after by many servants in the tradition of the nineteenth century. The house was destroyed by German bombs during the Second World War.

A house of an entirely different character was built in the north-east part of the park. It was not one of the 'Nash' villas built in the classical style. It was the Master's House of St Katherine's Hospital, which for centuries had been on a site near the Tower of London. In 1825–26, St Katherine's Hospital and the Master's House were moved away from the City of London and rebuilt in Regent's Park to designs prepared by the architect Ambrose Poynter. The hospital, with residential accommodation, was established on the east side of the Outer Circle, and the Master's House, built of plain brick in the Tudor style, was on the opposite side of the road. It was a large house, with gardens and stabling, but the style was foreign to John Nash's ideals and there is no doubt that he disapproved of the project. St Katherine's Hospital survived the Second World War but the Master's House was destroyed by a German missile. After the war the ground was restored to parkland and there is nothing left to indicate where the house stood.

Since the turn of the twentieth century, six new villas have been built for the Crown Commissioners at the north-west edge of the park, between the Outer Circle and the Regent's Canal.

The terraces

Apart from the glorious open spaces, the terraces are the most distinctive feature of Regent's Park. Unlike most of the individual villas already described, the terraces all survive, though in most cases with much modification internally and sometimes total reconstruction necessitated by serious decay. All invested with painted stucco, the terraces enliven the park with their external grandeur and elegant facades. In nearly all the houses, however, the interiors are plain, conforming to what became the standard pattern of domestic architecture in the Georgian and Regency periods.

Nash planned for thirteen terraces of houses to be built around the perimeter of the park. The terraces would face inwards towards the centre of the park, on the outer side of the drive that would encircle the park, the Outer Circle. They were designed to have an outward show of elegance, enhanced by stucco painted to simulate Portland stone.

When most of the terraces had been completed or were under construction, the Crown Commissioners decided to cancel the erection of the final two terraces, Munster Terrace and Carrick Terrace, both of which were to have been in the northern sector of the park.

Each terrace was named after a royal personage or a place associated with the Crown. There follows a list of those that were built, ranged clockwise round the perimeter of the park: York Terrace and York Gate, Ulster Terrace, Cornwall Terrace, Clarence Terrace, Sussex Place (Figure 18), Hanover Terrace, Gloucester Gate, Cumberland Terrace, Chester Terrace, Cambridge Terrace, Cambridge Gate. Outside the confines of the Outer Circle, a small terrace called Kent Terrace and another known as Park Terrace were built near Park Road, behind Hanover Terrace. Park Crescent, Park Square and St Andrew's Place must also be included in the list.

Nash provided for entrances to the park to be made between certain of the terraces. In his first plan there was provision for an entrance at the north end of

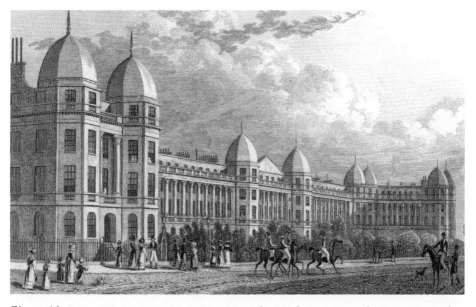

Figure 18 Sussex Place, a terrace designed by John Nash, in an unorthodox style, with views over the private gardens and the lake. It has been rebuilt and the houses are no longer in private occupation. From *London and Its Environs in the Nineteenth Century Illustrated by a Series of Views from Original Drawings by Thomas H. Shepherd* (London: James & Co., 1827).

Devonshire Place; but when the Marylebone parish church was re-sited on the Marylebone Road, close to the corner with the High Street, he altered his plan, to provide a more spectacular entrance facing the church. This was to become York Gate, and in the event it turned out to be one of Nash's most inspired achievements (Figure 10, page 26). Clockwise round the outer circle there were to be further entrances, namely: Clarence Gate, between Cornwall Terrace and Clarence Terrace; Hanover Gate; Macclesfield Gate, at the north end of Macclesfield Bridge over the canal near the zoo; Gloucester Gate (formerly East Gate), at the north-east corner of the park; Chester Gate, between Chester Terrace and Cambridge Terrace; and gates at Park Square East and Park Square West, leading from Park Crescent. Most of these gates were furnished with a keeper's lodge (Figure 19).

In a description of the various terraces, it is convenient to begin with York Terrace, if only because it embraces the most elegant entrance to the park. York Terrace is one of the largest terraces and among the most handsome. It was built in 1822, for the most part by the prodigious builder James Burton, owner of his own lakeside villa known as The Holme, already described. William Nurse collaborated in the building of the east half of the terrace. The facade was designed by Nash himself, who altered his first design by dividing the terrace into west and east halves in order to provide an entrance, York Gate, into the park between them. The two halves are symmetrical, initially comprising twenty

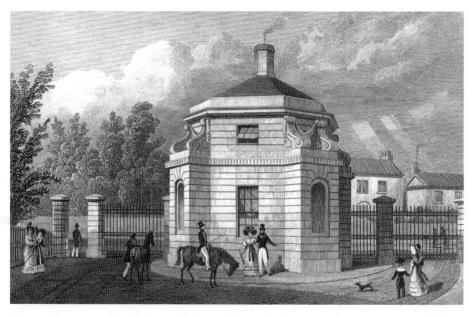

Figure 19 A typical gatekeeper's lodge, at Hanover Gate. It no longer stands. Close to its site now is the West London Mosque. From *London and Its Environs in the Nineteenth Century Illustrated by a Series of Views from Original Drawings by Thomas H. Shepherd* (London: James & Co., 1827).

houses in each part. In order to present a unified aspect as seen from the park, looking towards the Marylebone Road, Nash placed the entrances to the houses in the mews behind. Thus the facade seen from the park seems almost as if it were of a single palatial edifice. A separate building nearby comprises two individual houses but appears as one, known as the Doric Villa. Badly damaged in the Second World War, it was restored afterwards. The two main components of York Terrace are of four storeys, with Corinthian colonnades at ground-floor level surmounted by a continuous balcony. The central section of each half terrace projects forwards beyond the main parts, as do the extremes of the wings. A pediment on the central section is supported by six Ionic columns. The overall effect is truly elegant. In its heyday, in the middle of the nineteenth century, York Terrace was a favoured place of residence for the more wealthy members of the community, and for high ranking army officers in particular. The buildings were much damaged during the Second World War: after the war they were refurbished with radical alteration of the interiors to provide flats and other accommodation for students.

The term 'York Gate' comprises residential buildings as well as the gate itself, which closes off the park on the north side of Marylebone Road. The tall residential blocks, designed by Nash, stand on either side of the road leading into the park, a little to the south of York Terrace itself. These are elegant colonnaded buildings, so positioned that they enhance the stunning view obtained from the Outer Circle, with Hardwick's Marylebone parish church in the distance (Figure 10, page 26). They have now been adapted for commercial use.

A short walk along the Outer Circle brings the observer to the next terrace, named Cornwall Terrace, after the Dukedom of Cornwall, one of the Prince of Wales's titles. This was the first terrace to be built in the park, in 1821–22. It was designed by Decimus Burton when he was aged twenty-one. Nash gave his personal approval to the design, which was exhibited at the Royal Academy of Arts in 1822. The actual builder was James Burton, father of Decimus. The terrace consisted of nineteen houses, with front doors opening towards the park. The centre and the lateral wings extend forwards a little from the main body of the building and are furnished with Corinthian colonnades from the first to the second floors, surmounted with pediments. The end house on the north was given an elaborate bow window, lighting the ground floor and first floor, ornamented by four caryatids that form pilasters between the window frames. There being no provision for gardens, Decimus Burton suggested that an area in the park on the opposite side of the road should be railed off for the private use of the residents; but this idea was turned down by the Commissioners on the advice of John Nash. Cornwall Terrace had to be renovated after the Second World War on account of serious decay.

The next terrace along the Outer Circle, after Cornwall Terrace, is Clarence Terrace. Between these two terraces is Clarence Gate, which gives passage to Baker Street. A pretty lodge was designed by Nash, and wrought iron gates were made by John Peachy, a local ironsmith.

Clarence Terrace is the smallest of the major terraces. It was designed by Decimus Burton and built in 1823. Burton had to modify his original design to accommodate twelve houses instead of the original ten. There is a large central block with a pedimented Corinthian section in the middle, linked to forward-projecting lateral wings by an Ionic colonnade screening the two extra houses, which were made somewhat dark in consequence. From the terrace there are excellent views of the nearby lake. Clarence Terrace was in poor condition after the Second World War, and it was not possible to restore it. The facade was rebuilt to the original design, but the interior was refashioned to form flats.

There is only a driveway between Clarence Terrace and the next building, Sussex Place. As its name is different – 'Place' rather than 'Terrace' – so its architecture is entirely distinct. It was designed by John Nash himself and built in 1822 by William Smith, a wealthy builder responsible for work on several of the terraces. Distinguishing features of Sussex Place (see Figure 18) are its unusual shape – its wings are curved forwards, enclosing a space that was used for a private garden – and the ten pointed domes on the roof, which give it an Oriental appearance reminiscent of Nash's Regency Pavilion in Brighton. It is of similar length to Cornwall Terrace, and contained twenty-six houses, some with attractive spiral staircases. There are many three-sided bow windows, and between the windows at first- and second-floor levels are Corinthian columns, fifty-six in all. Although there was much adverse comment about Sussex Place soon after it was built, to modern eyes it has enormous charm. Furthermore, it is greatly enhanced by the superb views from the windows, more immediately of the private garden in front of the houses, and more distantly of the lake. Like so many of the Regent's Park terraces, Sussex Place suffered severely from decay, and after the Second World War it was found necessary to rebuild the facade and to remodel the interior for commercial use. Nevertheless, it remains an attractive feature of the park and a tribute to Nash's ingenuity.

Nash was also responsible for the design of Hanover Terrace (Figure 20), only a short distance along the Outer Circle from Sussex Place. The name is derived from the royal house of Hanover. The terrace was built more in the classical style of the period, and was rather 'up-market' compared with some of the other terraces. The frontage is handsome, with large pediments in the centre and at each end, each supported by four Doric columns. The ground floor is arcaded, with a railed balcony extending the whole length of the building. Each of the tall first-floor windows is pedimented. Gardens occupy the space between the houses and the road. Roof statues over the pediments – three over each – were much criticised and their removal was strongly recommended by, among others, James Elmes, the architect and author of *Metropolitan Improvements*, published in serial parts from 1827 onwards.

Owing to the cancellation of the building of the two terraces that Nash had planned for the north section of the park – Munster Terrace and Carrick Terrace – the next terraces are some distance away, beyond Gloucester Gate, which guards the route towards Camden Town. This gate is of architectural interest: it

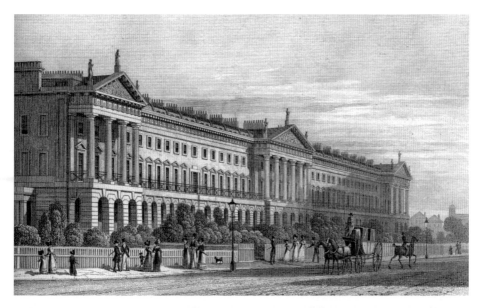

Figure 20 Hanover Terrace, named after the royal house of Hanover. It is one of the grandest terraces, with views over the lake and private gardens in front of the houses. From *London and Its Environs in the Nineteenth Century Illustrated by a Series of Views from Original Drawings by Thomas H. Shepherd* (London: James & Co., 1827).

consists of twin lodges with the driveway between them. The lodges were symmetrical, each with an arched-top window and a pediment pierced by a small oval window. The entablature was continued from the lodges across the roadway, supported between the lodges by two fluted Doric columns on each side. The whole effect is of a classical gem.

Next along the Outer Circle is a small terrace of houses known as Gloucester Gate, designed by John Scoles and built rather later than most of the terraces, in 1827. It has no special merit, but there was concern at the time because the architect deviated from Nash's preliminary sketch by enlarging the mouldings on the Corinthian columns, breaching the recognised convention.

Between Gloucester Gate and Cumberland Terrace was St Katherine's Hospital, transferred from its original ancient site near the Tower of London in 1825, as noted above. The new hospital was built with a central chapel separated from accommodation blocks on each side for the brothers and sisters. Opposite the hospital, on the other side of the Outer Circle, was the Master's House, already described, and demolished by enemy action during the Second World War. Almost uniquely in the park, these buildings were of plain brick construction, devoid of the stucco that Nash prescribed for his buildings.

Cumberland Terrace (Figure 21) was designed to be the superlative terrace, because in Nash's original design there was to be, facing it across the Outer Circle, a small palace for the Prince Regent. But the Regent had become King

George IV before the terrace was built, in 1826–27, and the palace never materialised. Cumberland Terrace is indeed a majestic building and must be regarded as John Nash's masterpiece. One of the longest terraces, it is composed of three separate sections, linked by high arches surmounted by statuary. The large central portion is colonnaded at the first and second storeys, with sixteen Corinthian pillars. The high pediment was furnished with three tall statues, and many further statues – not regarded as of high quality – adorned the high balcony above the second storey, the four elevated balconies adjacent to the two linking arches, and the balconies at the ends of the two wings. The ground floor was rusticated and subservient to the principal (first) floor. Gardens separate the houses from the road in front. There was a separate building – Cumberland Place – close to the end of the right wing of the terrace.

Chester Terrace, next on the Outer Circle to Cumberland Terrace, was less grandiose, even though largely designed by Nash himself. (He was perhaps in a hurry and neglectful, at a time when he was preoccupied with work for the King on Buckingham Palace.) This was one of the last terraces to be built (1825–26), and the builder again was James Burton. It is a long terrace, with a frontage of 900 feet. The straight outline is broken in the centre by a colonnade of eight Corinthian pillars, and there are similar but smaller colonnades in the middle

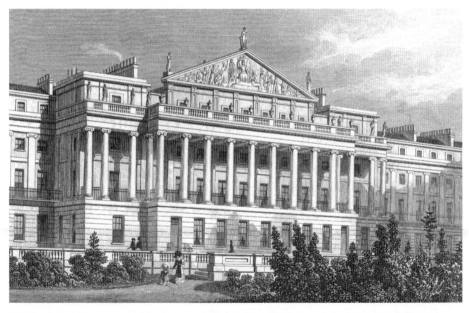

Figure 21 The central section of Cumberland Terrace, the largest terrace in Regent's Park and one of John Nash's masterpieces. It was designed in lavish style because the original intention had been to build, facing it, a small palace for the Prince Regent. From *London and Its Environs in the Nineteenth Century Illustrated by a Series of Views from Original Drawings by Thomas H. Shepherd* (London: James & Co., 1827).

and end of each wing, making five in total. The ground-floor and first-floor windows were tall but plain. An unbroken balcony extended along the whole length of the building at first-floor level. Individual double houses were built in front of each end of the terrace, separated from it by the driveway to the terrace. It seems that these houses were intended at first to form forward-projecting extremities of the terrace proper, rather than being isolated units. There was strong criticism of the layout at the time, with assertions that the houses in front were out of place and blocked the view from the end houses in the terrace. Nash tried to improve the situation by linking the houses to the main body of the terrace by triumphal arches; but critics remained disappointed. They also disliked the series of statues that had been placed above the parapet. In the end these were removed. This was a troublesome terrace, but it is still a great asset to the park. An interesting feature, too, is that there is a bust of John Nash on the outside of the southernmost part of the terrace, close to the exit to Albany Street, known as Chester Gate.

Cambridge Terrace was built as a plain and rather unattractive terrace of minor proportions, with three porticoes supported by ugly rusticated columns. It comprised only twelve houses. It was adjacent to the huge building to be described below, the Colosseum. When that building was pulled down in 1875, the Victorian block known as Cambridge Gate was erected on its site. This building, standing back from the road, has no great architectural or historical merit.

Adjacent to Cambridge Gate was a square building known as the Adult Orphan Asylum, a refuge for deprived women. Though designed by Nash, it was a rather plain building, later called Someries House when it became a private residence. It was demolished after the Second World War to make way for a fine modern building housing the Royal College of Physicians.

Adjacent to Someries House (to the south) was a short cul-de-sac known as St Andrew's Place, built in 1823–24, with two stylish houses at the far end and a small terrace of houses on the south side. On the north side is the lecture theatre of the Royal College of Physicians, with its curiously shaped non-vertical south wall. St Andrew's Place backs onto Park Square East, at right angles to it. At the other side of Park Square, adjoining the west side (Park Square West), is a matching terrace of attractive bow-fronted houses known as Ulster Terrace, built in 1824.

This completes the review of the terraces on the perimeter of the park, for Ulster Terrace is adjacent to York Terrace, already described.

The Zoological Gardens

London Zoo dates from the time that Regent's Park was being formed. There was no Zoological Society until the idea of forming one was put forward in 1824 by Sir Stamford Raffles, a colonial governor noted for having secured the island of Singapore, where the Raffles Hotel is still a prominent landmark. Fellows of the Royal Society, notably its President, Sir Humphry Davy, supported the scheme, and the Zoological Society of London was founded in April 1826, with Raffles as its first President. He had achieved his objective, but he had only a short tenure of office, for he died in the same year.

The aim of the Society, once formed, was to find a site on which to establish gardens in which to study and display animals, birds and other fauna. They approached the Crown Commissioners with a request to lease land in Regent's Park, preferably in the Inner Circle. This was not possible because land in the Inner Circle had already been committed to a nursery gardener. Instead they were offered five acres in the north-east section of the park, alongside the canal. They had requested twenty acres, and before long the extra land was granted, forming a triangular site adjacent to the canal and on both sides of the Outer Circle.

Fellows of the Society lost little time in developing the site for the reception of animals. Decimus Burton was instructed, and he submitted a suggested layout. His plan was not accepted in its entirety, but his general layout, and his designs for animals' quarters, including a camel house and a clock tower, were executed, and the Zoological Gardens were opened to Fellows of the Society in April 1828. A royal charter was granted in 1829, in which the aims of the Society were set down: 'The advancement of zoology and animal physiology, and the intro-duction of new and curious subjects of the Animal Kingdom'. The Society also had premises in Bruton Street, London, where there was a library, with meeting rooms and museum. The museum was closed in 1855, when the exhibits and specimens were transferred to the British Museum and other museums. A farm had also been acquired in Richmond, but it remained in the care of the Society only until 1834. Thereafter there was no country branch until Whipsnade Zoo near Dunstable, Bedfordshire, was opened in 1931.

At first the public were admitted to the Gardens only with a letter from a Fellow of the Society, and upon payment of the entry fee of one shilling. The requirement for a Fellow's letter was later relaxed: one shilling was still charged for admission, but for many years admission was restricted to Fellows on Sundays (later Sunday mornings only). The annual subscription for Fellows was at first two guineas and this was unchanged for many years. At the inception of the Society there were 151 Fellows, but the number grew rapidly, to over 1,000 within four years. In 1991 there were 2,225 Fellows.

The animals brought in for the opening of the Gardens were mostly gifts from various sources. The newspapers made much of the opening, reporting that the animals on display included monkeys, foxes, goats, beavers, emus, bears, llamas, gazelles, zebras and jackals. The first elephant arrived later in 1828. The collection was augmented in 1830 by the transfer of the menagerie from Windsor, and again in 1932 by animals from the Tower of London. The first chimpanzee was acquired in 1837 but he survived for only six months. There was greater success with giraffes, acquired in 1836: by 1839 they had already bred in captivity, and they continued to breed in the succeeding years. In 1840 a lion and lioness were brought from Tunis, but the lioness died after an accident and her mate pined for her and died a few weeks later. Other animals were acquired gradually. The Tsar of Russia presented two bison in 1847. The first hippopotamus came in 1850 and the first orang-utan in 1851. In 1876 the Prince of Wales (later Edward VII) brought a collection of animals from India; and similarly the next Prince of Wales (later King George V) presented another group of fauna, again from India, in 1912. These royal collections attracted large crowds of visitors: 900,000 were admitted in 1876, and 1,000,000 in 1912.

The first reptile house was built in 1843. There was an early tragedy when a keeper was bitten on the forehead by a cobra and died. The world's first aquarium was opened at the Zoo in 1853 and the first insect house in 1881. Another huge attraction was the first giant panda, which arrived in 1938, sparking a torrent of panda soft toys in the shops.

Meanwhile, there were repeated additions to the accommodation for the animals, birds, reptiles and other fauna. Decimus Burton designed a tunnel under the Outer Circle, simplifying access between the south and north sections of the gardens. The tunnel is still in use. Other architects were also instructed, notably Anthony Salvin (1799–1881), who, like Decimus Burton, had been a pupil of John Nash. Among other additions, Salvin was responsible for a new elephant house in 1868. As early as 1845, open-air terraces had been built for lions, tigers and other carnivores. In 1913, redesigned terraces for large animals were presented by J. Newton Mappin.

In more recent years, from the 1960s and 1970s, there have been huge, multi-million-pound developments, amounting to large-scale remodelling and reconstruction of the Gardens, under the direction of Sir Hugh Casson, one-time President of the Royal Academy, and F. A. P. Stengelhofen, the Society's architect. Notable also was the construction in 1963–64 of the huge aviary designed by Lord Snowdon. The Society's administrative departments on the Outer Circle were also extended, with the formation of an up-to-date, well equipped hospital for animals, the Nuffield Institute of Comparative Medicine and the Wellcome Institute of Comparative Physiology. These radical improvements have transformed London Zoo into one of the foremost such institutions in the world.

The Colosseum

During the fifty years of its existence, the Colosseum was a hugely prominent feature of Regent's Park and indeed of the whole area, visible from afar because of its enormous size and high domed roof.

The Colosseum was conceived by an enthusiastic surveyor, Thomas Horner, who lived in Robert Street, to the east of the park. Horner had spent many months perched each day in a small cabin on the top of the dome of St Paul's Cathedral, which was being repaired at the time. His objective was to make a series of drawings to show a panorama of London as seen from every angle. His lofty position allowed him to gain an uninterrupted view of the whole city. The only obstacle was the horrible pollution of the atmosphere, caused by smoke from innumerable domestic fires and industrial furnaces. To obviate this as far as possible, he started work at first light in the mornings, when the air was a little clearer. He is reported to have made more than 2,000 drawings when he completed his task in about 1822.

Horner next determined to promote the erection of a large building in which to display a panorama of London in paintings made from his drawings. In his words, he was 'determined to erect a permanent building for my panorama of London on a scale of unprecedented magnitude'. The intention was that the exhibition should be commercially viable, the public being invited to view the display for an entry fee of one shilling. Horner was a man of only moderate means, but he was able to enlist a sponsor prepared to gamble on the success of the venture.

Decimus Burton was the architect chosen to design the building, and John Nash gave his approval. Nash did, however, require Burton to scale down the size of the proposed building, which even so was enormous, as the name Colosseum suggests. It was a circular building (actually a sixteen-sided polygon) 130 feet in diameter, with a huge pillared portico and a domed roof 112 feet high at the apex. The portico, raised on a platform some feet from the ground, was vast, the frontage being equal to more than half the diameter of the rotunda itself. It was fronted by six massive Doric columns and surmounted by a handsome pediment (Figure 22).

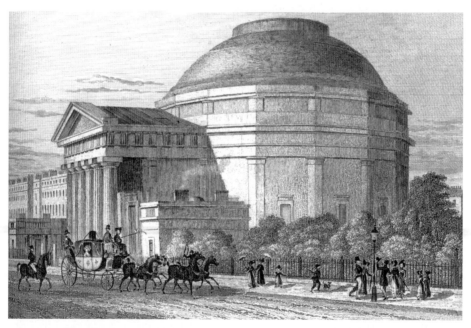

Figure 22 The Colosseum, a huge exhibition hall designed by Decimus Burton and built in 1825–27. Though a famous local attraction, it was financially insecure, and it was demolished in 1855. From *London and Its Environs in the Nineteenth Century Illustrated by a Series of Views from Original Drawings by Thomas H. Shepherd* (London: James & Co., 1827).

Construction of the building was completed in 1827, and it had been hoped that it would be opened to the public in the same year. But this was impossible because the artist – E. T. Parris – who had been commissioned to paint the panorama of London onto canvas from the drawings prepared by Thomas Horner was a long way from having completed the task. He had another year's work ahead, for it turned out that when he had finished he had covered 40,000 square feet of canvas. In the meantime, Thomas Horner, the originator of the project, and his sponsor had absconded, leaving debts of £60,000.

Despite this and other setbacks, the Colosseum was eventually opened to the public early in 1829. It was a fine building, surrounded by pleasant gardens and a small cottage nearby. The panorama of London was displayed in two galleries near the base of the dome; and above the galleries, at the very top of the building, was a viewing gallery, where, from its circumference, the visitor could see the real London in every direction.

To prevent frail visitors from suffering undue fatigue in climbing to the top of the building, a novel device was installed. This was one of the earliest lifts (perhaps the very first) to be installed in London. It was operated by a hydraulic mechanism, with an alternative hand-cranking facility as a standby.

The Colosseum proved to be a popular attraction but it was not a financial success. In 1831 it was bought as a speculative venture by John Braham, a famous tenor singer who had made a fortune in the previous thirty years, in conjunction with Frederick Henry Yates, an actor-manager with major theatre interests in London. Additions were made to the site, with the construction of two marine caverns and a so-called African glen, sporting a variety of stuffed animals. Also constructed was a large hall at the rear of the rotunda, with an entrance from Albany Street. (Houses in Colosseum Terrace, Albany Street, now mark the site.) The hall was finely decorated, with mirrored panels in the walls, bird-life paintings by a well known artist, and many reproductions of antique statues. It seems that little expense was spared. The hall was used not only for concerts but also for receptions, meetings and other functions associated with a certain amount of dressing up and pre-Victorian glamour. Later, in about 1838, it went down-market and was used more as a refreshment room and drinking bar. Even this did not shore up the finances: Braham's and Yates's investment proved an unmitigated disaster. In 1843 the building was sold to David Montague for 23,000 guineas – little more than half the amount that had been paid for it twelve years earlier. Under the new owner it was expensively refurbished. The artist E. T. Parris was brought back to repaint the panorama of London and to create a new panorama showing London by night. The whole site was revamped, with the construction of a Swiss chalet and classical ruins in the grounds. The new Colosseum was opened in 1845, with a private view for Queen Victoria and the Prince Consort. But three years later it was still faltering, and it was not saved by the staging of a cyclorama – a dramatic re-enactment of the huge earthquake that had rocked Lisbon in 1755. A revival for the Great Exhibition of 1851 also failed to cover the increasing debts, and the Colosseum was closed in 1855. There were no takers when it was offered for sale: it stood empty and decaying until 1875, when it had to be demolished.

The Diorama

The Colosseum was not the only site in Regent's Park that set out to provide an unusual spectacle for London audiences. Only a few dozen yards away was the Diorama, housed in the middle of Park Square East (Figure 23), the short terrace in the south-east corner of the park, adjacent to the New Road (Marylebone Road).

The Diorama was the invention of Louis Jacques Mandé Daguerre (1787–1851), a Frenchman who had been apprenticed to a scene designer at the Paris Opera and had later worked with Pierre Prévost, a master of the art of panorama. In 1816 Daguerre had turned to stage design and became famous for his brilliant lighting effects, notably for a special production of Aladdin in Paris. This work led him to the idea of diorama, a term that he formed from the Greek words *dia* (through) and *orama* (view, seeing).

A diorama might be described as an exhibition of very large paintings, usually of landscape, architectural features or places of special interest, enlivened by skilful manipulation of the lighting and other devices. Light was projected on to

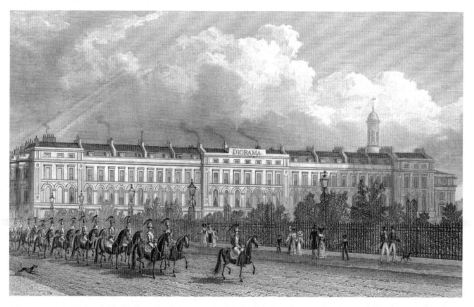

Figure 23 Park Square East, the central section of which housed the Diorama, where huge pictures were shown illuminated in such a way as to give a lifelike effect. It was the invention of Louis Jacques Mandé Daguerre, one of the pioneers of photography. From *London and Its Environs in the Nineteenth Century Illustrated by a Series of Views from Original Drawings by Thomas H. Shepherd* (London: James & Co., 1827).

the picture from the front or from behind. Rear lighting allowed images painted on the back of the translucent canvas to be seen from the front. Shutters and mirrors controlled the light, and tinted screens allowed a certain amount of colour to be introduced. It might even be possible to give an impression of movement by manipulation of artefacts behind the picture, for instance by the emission of real smoke. By such means remarkably lifelike effects could be created. Thus, a painting of a room that appeared to be empty when illuminated from the front might appear to be full of people when lit from behind to display images painted on the back of the canvas. Or a building that seemed to be in good order when lit from the front might be seen to be suddenly in flames when lit from behind through an orange-coloured screen, and licked by smoke created close to the picture.

The technique of producing such effects was clearly very demanding of the operator's skill, and experienced operators were required. Daguerre himself was a master of such detail, and together with his associate, Charles-Marie Bouton (1786–1853), he had established the first diorama in Paris in 1822, with such success that he was encouraged to bring a similar project to London.

A diorama needed a special building, because the pictures to be shown were very large (thirty feet or more across) and had to be viewed at a distance, from a darkened location. The design of the Paris Diorama was brought to London, where the construction of houses in Park Square East was just beginning. John Nash agreed to the design submitted by Daguerre. He himself designed the front elevation of the terrace, but the Diorama building behind the centre of the terrace became the responsibility of Augustus Charles Pugin, one of Nash's associates, who was assisted by an engineer, James Morgan.

The design was largely a copy of the Diorama in Paris. The core of the building was a huge cylinder, thirty-nine feet in diameter and twenty-five feet high. This was to house the circular, rotating auditorium, a unique feature of the Diorama, made necessary by the planned technique of exhibiting two huge pictures in fairly rapid succession. Daguerre postulated that instead of changing the pictures after the first one had been shown, it was easier to leave the pictures in position and to move the audience to face the second picture. This explains the cylindrical design of the building and the circular auditorium, which was free to rotate round a fixed central pivot, running smoothly on rails. It was said that the auditorium and the audience of 200 people, a total weight of perhaps twenty tons, could easily by moved by one person, so efficient was the mechanism devised by James Morgan. The concept of a revolving auditorium had worked well in the Paris Diorama, so it was repeated in the Regent's Park model.

In actual fact there was only a partial revolution of the auditorium, through seventy-three degrees. This was sufficient to allow the audience to face, in turn, two dark tunnels, at the ends of which the illuminated pictures were displayed. After the first picture had been shown, the auditorium was moved round through the arc of seventy-three degrees, to bring the second picture into view (see Figure 24).

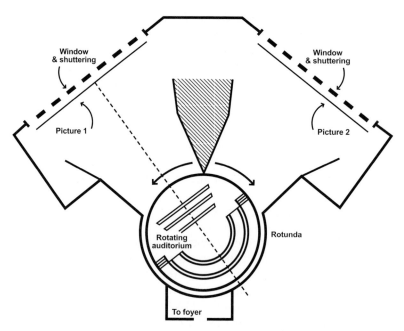

Figure 24 Plan of the Regent's Park Diorama at the level of the auditorium. Large pictures, suitable illuminated, were mounted at the ends of each of two wide tunnels, to be viewed by the audience from a distance. When the first picture had been shown, the circular auditorium, with the seated audience, was swivelled through about seventy-three degrees, to face the second picture at the end of the second tunnel. Only two pictures were shown at each session. Because of the need to manipulate the lighting of each of the two huge pictures to produce life-like effects, it was found easier to move the audience between the two showings, rather than to move the pictures.

The Diorama in Regent's Park was completed in four months, at a cost of £9,000. It was opened to the public in September 1823. It became a conspicuous landmark, for large capital letters high up on the parapet spelt out the word DIORAMA. Visitors to the exhibition, upon their arrival in the auditorium, were treated to a foretaste of what was to come: light from the ceiling, softened by a semi-transparent fabric, illuminated a series of panels containing portraits of great painters of the past and present. The exhibition of the pictures themselves occupied only half an hour, for an entrance fee of one shilling, later raised to two shillings – a substantial charge at the time.

Among the first pictures to be shown at the Diorama were two that had been popular when shown in Paris a year before. These were *The Valley of Surnen, Switzerland*, painted by Daguerre himself, and *The Chapel of the Trinity, Canterbury Cathedral*, by Charles Bouton. Published reviews (possibly prompted by the publicity-conscious Daguerre) were 'ecstatic'. One critic described Bouton's depiction of the interior of Trinity Chapel in Canterbury as follows:

the whole is at one moment subdued by gloom, seeming to be caused by the intervention of a passing cloud ... until the place becomes awfully imposing; when, in an instant, as though the interruption had passed away, and the sun was permitted to shine through the windows in its full lustre, the Gothic architecture is beautifully illumined.

About the Swiss landscape the critic enthused with continuing hyperbole:

The scene undergoes similar changes, in which the bursts of sunshine are admirably executed, and particularly in the effects produced in the sky and on the clouds, which continually seem to form new combinations of light, colour and arrangement.

Subsequent pictures, mostly shipped from the Diorama in Paris, continued the themes of romantic Alpine landscapes, Gothic ruins and such relics as Fountain's Abbey in Yorkshire; and there were travel scenes with depiction of favourite sites in Paris, or Italian monuments. More topically, in 1839 the Diorama exhibited a painting by Bouton depicting the coronation of Queen Victoria.

The success of the Diorama was heavily dependent upon the quality of the pictures, which were changed only every three to six months – hardly often enough to keep people coming. Success also required the retention of skilled operators to handle the presentation and lighting, to ensure maximum impact upon the audience. These factors in turn depended upon the work that Daguerre and Bouton put into the project. It proved difficult for them to keep up with the task of producing new pictures, to maintain interest.

After leaving London in 1830, seven years after the Diorama opened, Daguerre concentrated his interest in the development of photography, leaving Bouton in London to run the Diorama. Inevitably, attendances dwindled, and the Diorama was sold in 1839, when Bouton, too, returned to Paris. New management failed to revive interest and the project ended in 1850. The building was bought by Sir Samuel Morton Peto, a Member of Parliament and a devout Baptist. He converted it in Byzantine style and it became the Regent's Park Chapel. His name was given to Peto Place, the mews behind the terrace. Later, the building housed the Arthur Stanley Institute for Rheumatic Disease, a department of the Middlesex Hospital, with a detachment of the school of physiotherapy. After total refurbishment in the 1990s it was taken over by the Prince's Trust, a charity founded in 1976 by the Prince of Wales, dedicated to improving the lives of underprivileged young people in the United Kingdom.

The Inner Circle

John Nash had originally recommended that there should be a double circus, each circus lined by terraces of houses, situated eccentrically near the middle of the park. But the Commissioners disallowed this, and a single circular driveway, without terraces of houses, was constructed. The ground within the circle was left open, and much of it was rented out at first to a garden nurseryman. In 1839, when the Royal Botanic Society was founded, eighteen acres of land were leased to it. Elaborate gardens were laid out by Robert Marnock under the direction of the long-term Secretary, James de Carle Sowerby. In addition to the many beds and herbaceous borders, there was a large conservatory, with a museum of plant specimens, and a library. Also within the Inner Circle, from 1846 to 1861, was an observatory built for George Bishop, the first tenant of nearby South Villa (see above).

Open-air theatre

At various times, plays were staged in the Inner Circle from about 1900 onwards. Shakespeare's *Twelfth Night* and *A Midsummer Night's Dream* were always popular. In June 1933 a theatre was formally opened in the north-west sector of the Inner Circle, with a fresh production of *Twelfth Night* directed by Robert Atkins. Shakespeare's plays produced by the New Shakespeare Company were generally successful. Ballet and opera were staged occasionally. In 1972–75 the open-air theatre was totally reconstructed, to provide traditional seating for audiences of 1,200.

Queen Mary's Gardens

When the Royal Botanic Society was disbanded in 1931, after a profitable life of nearly a century, care of the gardens was taken over by the Royal Parks Division of the Ministry of Public Building and Works. The conservatory was taken down and some of the trees were felled. The Polygon Restaurant, made up from multiple hexagonal units, now stands where the Society had its offices.

The gardens were well tended in their new form. The rosary was enlarged and replanted with hundreds of new bushes. In 1932, in honour Queen Mary, who had for a long time shown a keen interest, the gardens were named after her, as Queen Mary's Gardens. Alongside the rose garden is a small lake, the home of many species of water fowl. Close by is the Mound, a large hillock formed from soil excavated when the Regent's Park Lake was dug out. It features a colourful display of plants and shrubs, and a path winding to the top. In the shelter of the Mound are a rock garden and a roaring artificial waterfall rushing into the lake. Entrance to Queen Mary's Gardens from the driveway of the Inner Circle is through gilded wrought iron gates presented by Sigismund Goetze, a notable artist who lived in one of the Nash villas, and a generous benefactor of the Marylebone area.

Other gardens within the park

St John's Garden, already mentioned, was formed as the private garden of St John's Lodge, the villa built near the west side of the Inner Circle. After 1889, when the villa was acquired by the third Marquess of Bute, the garden was lovingly restored and planted with many varieties of trees and shrubs. The garden, separated from the villa, is now open to the public and is approached through a path directly from the Inner Circle. It is a haven of peace and quiet, beloved by those who like to get away for a time from the cares of the world.

Broad Walk is an attractive feature of the park, laid out by John Nash. It continues the line of Portland Place, extending northwards across the park from Park Square to rejoin the Outer Circle close to the zoo. The southern half of the Walk is lined on each side by large flower beds, interspersed by huge stone urns, all planted with appropriate plants throughout the year. Halfway along this part of the Walk is the well known Dolphin Fountain, by Alexander Munro (1852). Formerly in Hyde Park, the fountain was brought here in the 1960s. The Broad Walk in Regent's Park must be classed as one of the most beautiful pathway gardens in Britain.

Appendix

Lister's 1867 paper on antisepsis

Over a century and a half after the full acceptance of Lister's work, it is instructive again to read his historic original paper. There follows the text of the paper that was published in *The Lancet* of 16 March 1867, with the rather lengthy title 'On a new method of treating compound fracture, abscess, etc., with observation on the conditions of suppuration'.

The frequency of disastrous consequences in compound fracture, contrasted with the complete immunity from danger to life or limb in simple fracture, is one of the most striking as well as melancholy facts in surgical practice.

If we inquire how it is that an external wound communicating with the seat of fracture leads to such grave results, we cannot but conclude that it is by inducing, through access to the atmosphere, decomposition of the blood which is effused in greater or less amount around the fragments and among the interstices of the tissues, and, losing by putrefaction its natural bland character, and assuming properties of an acrid irritant, occasions both local and general disturbance.

We know that blood kept exposed to the air at the temperature of the body, in a vessel of glass or other material chemically inert, soon decomposes; and there is no reason to suppose that the living tissues surrounding a mass of extravasated blood could preserve it from being affected in a similar manner by the atmosphere. On the contrary, it may be ascertained as a matter of observation that, in a compound fracture, twenty-four hours after the accident the coloured serum which oozes from the wound is already distinctly tainted with the odour of decomposition, and during the next two or three days, before suppuration has set in, the smell of the effused fluids becomes more and more offensive.

This state of things is enough to account for all the bad consequences of the injury.

The pernicious influence of decomposing animal matter upon the tissues has probably been under-rated, in consequence of the healthy state in which granulating sores remain in spite of a very offensive condition of their discharges. To argue from this, however, that fetid material would be innocuous in a recent wound would be to make a great mistake. The granulations being composed of an imperfect form of tissue, insensible and indisposed to absorption, but with remarkably active cell development, and perpetually renovated as fast as it is destroyed at the surface, form a most admirable protective layer, or living plaster. But before a raw surface has granulated, an acrid discharge acts with unrestrained effect upon it, exciting the sensory nerves, and causing through them both local inflammation and general fever, and also producing by its caustic action a greater or less extent of sloughs, which must be thrown off by a corresponding suppuration, while there is at the same time a risk of absorption of the poisonous fluids into the circulation.

This view of the cause of the mischief in compound fracture is strikingly corroborated by cases in which the external wound is very small. Here, if the coagulum at the orifice is allowed to dry and form a crust, as was advised by John Hunter, all bad consequences are probably averted, and, the air being excluded, the blood beneath becomes organised and absorbed, exactly as in a simple fracture. But if any accidental circumstance interferes with the satisfactory formation of the scab, the smallness of the wound, instead of being an advantage, is apt to prove injurious, because, while decomposition is permitted, the due escape of foul discharge is prevented. Indeed, so impressed are some surgeons with the evil which may result from this latter cause, that, deviating from the excellent Hunterian practice, they enlarge the orifice with the knife in the first instance and apply fomentations, in order to mitigate the suppuration which they render inevitable.

Turning now to the question how the atmosphere produces decomposition of organic substances, we find that a flood of light has been thrown upon this most important subject by the philosophic researches of M. Pasteur, who has demonstrated by thoroughly convincing evidence that it is not to its oxygen or to any of its gaseous constituents that the air owes this property, but to minute particles suspended in it, which are the germs of various low forms of life, long since revealed by the microscope, and regarded as merely accidental concomitants of putrescence, but now shown by Pasteur to be its essential cause, resolving the complex organic compounds into substances of simpler chemical constitution, just as the yeast-plant converts sugar into alcohol and carbonic acid.

A beautiful illustration of this doctrine seems to me to be presented in surgery by pneumothorax with emphysema, resulting from puncture of the lung by a fractured rib. Here, though atmospheric air is perpetually introduced into the pleura in great abundance, no inflammatory disturbance supervenes; whereas an external wound penetrating the chest, if it remains open, infallibly causes dangerous suppurative pleurisy. In the latter case the blood and serum poured out into the pleural cavity, as an immediate consequence of the injury, are decomposed by the germs that enter with the air, and then operate as a powerful irritant upon the serous membrane. But in case of puncture of the lung without external wound, the atmospheric gases are filtered of the causes of decomposition before they enter the pleura, by passing through the bronchial tubes, which, by their small size, their tortuous course, their mucous secretion, and ciliated epithelial lining, seem to be specially designed to arrest all solid particles in the air inhaled. Consequently the effused fluids retain their original character unimpaired, and are speedily absorbed by the unirritated pleura.

Applying these principles to the treatment of compound fracture, bearing in mind that it is from the vitality of the atmospheric particles that all the mischief arises, it appears that all that is requisite is to dress the wound with some material capable of killing these septic germs, provided that any substance can be found reliable for this purpose, yet not too potent as a caustic.

In the course of the year 1864 I was much struck with an account of the remarkable effects provided by carbolic acid upon the sewage of the town of Carlisle, the admixture of a very small proportion not only preventing all odour from the lands irrigated with the refuse material, but, as it was stated, destroying the entozoa which usually infest cattle fed upon such pastures.

My attention having for several years been much directed to the subject of suppuration, more especially in its relation to decomposition, I saw that such a powerful antiseptic was peculiarly adapted for experiments with a view to elucidating that subject, and while I was engaged in the investigation the applicability of carbolic acid for the treatment of compound fracture naturally occurred to me.

My first attempt of this kind was made in the Glasgow Royal Infirmary in March, 1865, in a case of compound fracture of the leg. It proved unsuccessful, in consequence, as I now believe, of improper management; but subsequent trials have more than realised my most sanguine anticipations.

Carbolic acid proved in various ways well adapted for the purpose. It exercises a local sedative influence upon the sensory nerves; and hence is not only almost painless in its immediate action on a raw surface, but speedily renders a wound entirely free from uneasiness. When employed in compound fracture its caustic properties are mitigated so as to be unobjectionable by admixture with the blood, with which it forms a tenacious mass that hardens into a dense crust, which long retains its antiseptic virtue, and has other advantages, as will appear from the following cases, which I will relate in the order of their occurrence, premising that as the treatment has been gradually improved, the earlier ones are not to be taken as patterns.

Case 1. James G—, aged 11 years, was admitted into Glasgow Royal Infirmary on August 12th, 1865, with compound fracture of the left leg, caused by the wheel of an empty cart passing over the limb a little below its middle. The wound, which was about an inch and a half long, and three-quarters of an inch broad, was close to, but not exactly over, the line of the fracture of the tibia. A probe, however, could be passed beneath the integument over the seat of fracture and for some inches beyond it. Very little blood had been extravasated into the tissues. My house surgeon, Dr Macfee, acting under my instructions, laid a piece of lint dipped in liquid carbolic acid upon the wound, and applied lateral paste-board splints padded with cotton wool, the limb resting on its outer side, with the knee bent. It was left undisturbed for four days, when, the boy complaining of some uneasiness, I removed the inner splint and examined the wound. It showed no signs of suppuration, but the skin in its immediate vicinity had a slight blush of redness. I now dressed the sore with lint soaked with water having a small proportion of carbolic acid diffused through it; and this was continued for five days, during which the uneasiness and the redness of the skin disappeared, the sore meanwhile furnishing no pus, although some superficial sloughs caused by the acid were separating. But the epidermis being excoriated by this dressing, I substituted for it a solution of one part of carbolic acid in from ten to twenty parts of olive oil, which was used for four days, during which a small amount of imperfect pus was produced from the surface of the sore, but not a drop appeared from beneath the skin. It was now clear that there was no longer any danger of deep-seated suppuration, and simple water dressing was employed. Cicatrisation proceeded just as in an ordinary granulating sore. At the expiration of six weeks I examined the condition of the bones, and, finding them firmly united, discarded the splints: and two days later the sore was entirely healed, so that the cure could not be said to have been at all retarded by the circumstance of the fracture being compound.

This, no doubt, was a favourable case, and might have done well under ordinary treatment. But the remarkable retardation of suppuration, and the immediate conversion of the compound fracture into a simple fracture with a superficial sore, were most encouraging facts.

This article is reprinted with permission from Elsevier, from Lister J. On a new method of treating compound fracture, abscess, etc. Part 1 On compound fracture. *The Lancet* March 16, 1867: 326–9. The article continues in the following issues: March 23, 1867: 357–9, March 30, 1867: 387–9 and April 27, 1867: 507–9.

Bibliography

Material for this book came mostly from published sources, some contemporary with the development of the Harley/Portland estate. I acknowledge my indebtedness to the following authors and publishers.

Ashford, E. B. (1960) *Lisson Green*. London: Marylebone Society.

Barton, N. (1992) *The Lost Rivers of London*. London: Historical Publications Ltd.

Blackham, R. J. (undated) *London, the Sovereign City*. London: Sampson Low.

Elmes, J. (1827) *Metropolitan Improvements; or London in the Nineteenth Century*. London: Jones & Co.

Howitt, W. (1869) *The Northern Heights of London*. London: Longmans, Green & Co.

Larwood, J. (1881) *The London Parks*. London: Chatto & Windus.

Mackenzie, G. (1972) *Marylebone*. London: Macmillan.

Pound, R. (1967) *Harley Street*. London: Michael Joseph.

Samuel, E. S. (1959) *The Villas in Regent's Park*. London: Marylebone Society.

Saunders, A. (1981) *Regent's Park*. London: Bedford College.

Shepherd, T. H. (1827) *London and Its Environs in the Nineteenth Century Illustrated by a Series of Views from Original Drawings by Thomas H. Shepherd*. London: James & Co.

Smith, T. (1833) *A Topographical and Historical Account of the Parish of St Mary-le-bone*. London: John Smith.

Summerson, J. (1945) *Georgian London*. London: Pleiades Books.

I have also relied upon material from the following journals: *Annals of the Royal Society of Medicine*; *British Journal of Surgery*; *British Medical Journal*; *Journal of Bone and Joint Surgery*; *The Lancet*.

Index

Page references to *figures and tables* are shown in *italics*.

Adam, Robert and James 13
Adams, Henry Brook (historian) 13
Adult Orphan Asylum (Someries House) 93
Albany Cottage, Regent's Park 83–4, *84*
All Souls, Langham Place 24, *25*
antiseptic surgery, Joseph Lister 39–40
Asquith, Herbert Henry, 1st Earl of Oxford
    and Asquith, Prime Minister 12

Bedford College, Regent's Park *81*, 82–3
Benson, Robert, Lord Bingley 11
Bentinck, Henry, 1st Duke of Portland 17
Bentinck, Lord George, statue 12
Bentinck, William, 2nd Duke of Portland
    17–18
Bentinck, William, 1st Earl of Portland 17
Bentinck, William Henry Cavendish, 3rd
    Duke of Portland 18
Bentinck-Scott, William Henry Cavendish,
    5th Duke of Portland 18
birth control *see* contraception
Bishop, George (President, Royal
    Astronomical Society) 83, 110
Bosanquet, William (banker) 29
Braham, John (tenor) 97
British Orthopaedic Association,
    founding 56
Brydges, James, 1st Duke of Chandos 10–11
Burnett, Frances Hodgson (author) 13
Burton, Decimus (architect) 80–6, 89–90,
    94–6

Cambridge Gate, Regent's Park *81*, 93
Cambridge Terrace, Regent's Park 87–8, 93
Campbell, Thomas, *Lord George Bentinck*
    12
Casson, Sir Hugh 95
Cavendish Square 9–12, *20*
    varying medical prestige 69
Chandos House 12, 60
Chester Terrace, Regent's Park 92–3
Clarence Gate, Regent's Park *81*, 88–9
Clarence Terrace, Regent's Park 89–90
clinical pathology 64
Clover, Joseph (anaesthetist) 33, 34
Colosseum, Regent's Park 95–8, *96*
contraception 62–3
Cornwall Terrace, Regent's Park 89
Cumberland Terrace, Regent's Park 91–2,
    92

Daguerre, Louis Jacques Mandé *98*,
    98–101
Dawson, Bertrand, 1st Viscount Dawson
    of Penn 61–3
de Grey, George, Lord Walsingham 29
de Vere, Robert, 2nd Earl of Oxford 5
Dean's Mews 12
Devonshire Place 15
Diorama, Regent's Park *98*, 98–101, *100*
Duke of Cumberland statue 12

early medical practices 31–2

Elphinstone, George Keith, 1st Viscount Keith 27
Epstein, Jacob, *Madonna and Child* 12

fading prestige 69–71
Fairbank, Sir Thomas 57–8
Foley House 12, 13
Fordyce, John (Surveyor General for Crown Lands in London) 74

Gibbs, James (architect) 19, 23
Gladstone, William E., Prime Minister 28
Gloucester Gate, Regent's Park *81*, 90–1
Godlee, Rickman John (surgeon) 51–2
Goetze, Sigismund (artist) 86, 102
Gordon, George, Lord 28–9
Greenough, George Bellas (geologist and geographer) 86
Grove House, Regent's Park *85*, 85–6

Hanover Gate, Regent's Park *81, 88*
Hanover Lodge, Regent's Park 84
Hanover Square 9–10
Hanover Terrace, Regent's Park 79, 90, *91*
Harcourt, Simon, 1st Viscount Harcourt 11
Harcourt House 11
Hardwick, Thomas (architect) 24, *26*
Harley, Edward, 2nd Earl of Oxford and Mortimer 7, 9
Harley, Edward (Knight of the Bath) 6
Harley, George, M.D.,F.R.S. 34
Harley, Margaret Cavendish, Lady 15
Harley, Richard de 6
Harley, Robert, 1st Earl of Oxford and Mortimer 6–7
Harley, Robert (Master of the Mint) 6
Harley Street
    area, plan 1746 *4*
    early medical practices 31–2
    fading prestige 69–71
    major construction 19–20
    multiple tenancies 67–8
    specialist medical practices 32–5
    today 68–9
    typical houses 20–3, *21*
Henrietta Street (Place) 10
Henry VIII, King 5

Hertford (St Dunstan's) Villa, Regent's Park 84–5
Hobson, Thomas 5
Holford House, Regent's Park 86
Holles, Henrietta Cavendish, Lady 6, 9
Holles, John, Duke of Newcastle 5–6
The Holme, Regent's Park *81*, 81–2, *82*
Holroyd, James, 1st Earl of Sheffield 13
Hood, Alexander, 1st Viscount Bridport 27
Horder, Thomas Jeeves, 1st **Baron Horder of Ashford** 63–5
Horner, Thomas (surveyor) 95–7
Horsley, Sir Victor 53
Horwood, Richard, *plan of London, 1792-99 14*
Howard de Walden estate 15
Huguenot refugees 3
Hunter, John (surgeon) 32
Hutchinson, Sir Jonathan (surgeon) 33

Inner Circle, Regent's Park 101–2
Islamic Cultural Centre, Regent's Park *81*, 84

James I, King 5, 6
Jew's Harp tea garden 73, 78
Jones, Sir Robert 56–7, 59

Lane, Sir William Arbuthnot 54–5
Langham Hotel 12
Lilestone Manor 5
Lisson Green 5
Lister, Joseph 37–50
    12 Park Crescent *38*
    antiseptic surgery 39–40
    early life 38–40
    life in Edinburgh 38
    life in Glasgow 38
    life in London 40–1
    modern appraisal of his techniques 49–50
    paper on antisepsis, 1867 105–9
    portrait *39*
    public memorials 41–9
Liston, Robert (surgeon) 37
Little, Muirhead 55–6
Long, Crawford 37

Long, John St John 31–2
Lyell, Sir Charles (geologist) 28

Macclesfield Gate, Regent's Park 88
Mackenzie, Sir Morell (laryngologist) 34–5
Madonna and Child, Jacob Epstein 12
Mappin, J. Newton (architect) 95
Marylebone, Borough (parish) of 5
  population 27
Marylebone Basin 3, 4, 13
Marylebone Fields 2–3, 4
Marylebone gardens 2–3, 4
Marylebone Park 5, 14, 74–6
Marylebone Road 3, 13–15, 24, 25, 78–9
Marylebone village 1–2, 4
Master's House, St Katherine's Hospital,
  Regent's Park 86
Milbanke, Sir Ralph 13
Morgan, James (architect) 75–6
Morton, William Thomas Green
  (physician) 37

Nash, John (architect) 13, 24, 25
  Regent's Park 75–80
National Health Service, introduction
  1948 70–1
New Road *see* Marylebone Road
Nightingale, Florence 28
Nuffield Institute of Comparative
  Medicine 81, 95

observatory, Regent's Park 83, 102
open-air theatre, Regent's Park 102
ophthalmology 60–1
orthopaedic surgery
  American assistance, WW1 56
  beginnings 55
  rapprochement with general surgery
    58–9
  struggle for recognition 56
Oxford Chapel 9, 10, 23
Oxford Market 23

Park Crescent, Regent's Park 79, 81, 88
Park Square, Regent's Park 78, 81, 93, 98, 99
Parris, Edmund Thomas (artist) 97
Pasteur, Louis 39

Pepys, Samuel 2
Pinero, Sir Arthur Wing 28
Portland, Dukes of 17–19
Portland estate 12, 13–15
Portland Place 13, 15
Portman estate 5
Prince, John (surveyor) 9
Pugin, Augustus Charles (architect) 99

Queen Mary's Gardens, Regent's Park 86,
  102
Queen's Head and Artichoke, Albany
  Street (tavern) 73, 78

Raffles, Sir Stamford 93–4
Ramsay, Allan, artist 27
Regent Street, inception 74, 77
Regent's canal 77–8, 81, 85–8, 94
Regent's Park
  Broad Walk 103
  Colosseum 95–8, 96
  Diorama 98, 98–101, 100
  early development 73–4
  Inner Circle 101–2
  Nash's plan 75–82, 81
  open-air theatre 102
  plan 81
  Queen Mary's Gardens 102
  Royal College of Physicians 81, 93
  St John's Garden 102–3
  terraces 79–80, 86–93
    Holme, 81, 81–2, 88
  villas 80–6
  York Gate 79, 89
  Zoological Gardens 79, 93–5
Repton, Humphry (landscape gardener) 75
Rocque, John, *plan Harley Street area,*
  1746 4
Rose of Normandy, tavern, Marylebone 2
Rose Tavern, Marylebone 2–3
Royal Botanic Society 102
Royal College of Physicians, Regent's Park
  81, 93
Royal Society of Medicine, 1 Wimpole
  Street 12, 60

Shepherd, Edward (architect) 10

Smith, Thomas, *A Topographical and Historical Account of the Parish of St. Mary-le-bone*, 1833 2, 11–12, *16*, 29
South Sea Company 7, 10
South Villa, Regent's Park 83, *83*
specialist medical practices 32–5
St Andrew's Place, Regent's Park 93
St Dunstan's (Hertford) Villa, Regent's Park 84–5
St John's Lodge, Regent's Park 82–3
St Mary, Marylebone 23–4, *24*, 79
St Marylebone Parish Church, Marylebone Road 24, *26*
St Mary-le-Bourn *see* Marylebone village
St Peter's, Vere Street *see* Oxford Chapel
Stengelhofen, F. A. P. 95
Still, Sir George Frederick 53
Sussex Place, Regent's Park *87*, 90
Syme, James (surgeon) 38

terraces, Regent's Park 79–80, 86–93
The Holme, Regent's Park *81*, 81–2, *82*
Thompson, Sir Henry 33–4
Trethowan, William (orthopaedic surgeon) 68

Treves, Sir Frederick 52–3
Trinity Church, Albany Street 24–5
Turk's Head, public house 23
Turner, Joseph Mallord William, artist 27
Tweedy, Sir John 60–1
Tyburn, Manor of 1, 5
Tyburn Road 1–2
Tyburn (Tybourn), stream 1

Upper Harley Street 15

Wellcome Institute of Comparative Physiology 95
Wellesley, Arthur, Lord Wellington 27
Wimpole Street 19, 52
    No.1 Royal Society of Medicine 12, 60
    today 68

York Gate, Regent's Park *26*, 79, 89
York Terrace, Regent's Park 88–9

Zoological Gardens, Regent's Park 79, 93–5